PRAISE FOR OZ GARCIA

D1311839

"Oz Garcia has done a terrific job of helping us all understand hormones play such an amazing role in keeping you healthy. This is a must-read for people committed to taking control of their health and wellness for life."
—Pamela M. Peeke, M.D., M.P.H., author of *Fight Fat After Forty*, assistant clinical professor of medicine, University of Maryland

"*Look and Feel Fabulous Forever* is a magical blend of nutrition, science, wonder, and hope. For all of us who want to feel twenty-five again—and look great while we're at it—Oz provides us with 'tomorrow's medicine today' complete with all the essential tools and resources for quality longevity and successful aging. You have in your hands an indispensable guide to your best body—ever!"
—Ann Louise Gittleman, author of *Before the Change* and *The Fat Flush Plan*

"*Look and Feel Fabulous Forever* weaves Oz Garcia's insights with the wisdom from the best minds in science and research to produce a terrific, user-friendly guide to optimum fitness."
—Ronald A. Ruden, M.D., Ph.D., author of *The Craving Brain*

"*Look and Feel Fabulous Forever* is required reading for all our patients as part of their facial rejuvenation process."
—Stephen Bosniak, M.D., and Marian Cantisano-Zilkha, M.D., facial cosmetic surgeons and authors of *Non-Invasive Techniques for Facial Rejuvenation*

"Oz Garcia brings energy and excitement to the field of nutrition that will motivate people to achieve greater health. Backed by solid research and years of experience, Oz Garcia's fresh and exciting approach makes this book a cutting-edge resource and great reading for all."
—Dr. Richard Firshein author of *The Nutraceutical Revolution*

"I'll always be a devoted fan and wish more people 'Oz health.' I'm miraculously healthier, more energetic, and more physically fit."
—Ellen Asmedeo, publisher and vice president, *Travel & Leisure* magazine

"Oz Garcia, is by far the most thorough, knowledgeable nutrition/body expert in New York, which in my opinion means the universe."
—Michelle Kessler, accessories editor, *Vogue*

"From the moment I committed to Oz Garcia's program, I immediately felt better and it was not only his eating and supplement game plan, but also his understanding and personal commitment to me."
—Rachel Hayes, beauty and fitness editor, *Cosmopolitan*

Look and Feel Fabulous Forever

The World's Best Supplements, Anti-Aging Techniques, and High-Tech Health Secrets

Oz Garcia

with Sharyn Kolberg

PREVIOUSLY PUBLISHED UNDER THE TITLE *OZ GARCIA'S THE HEALTHY HIGH-TECH BODY*

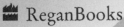

ReganBooks

An Imprint of HarperCollinsPublishers

To Clara and Osvaldo Garcia, my mother and father,
for the extraordinary and inspiring lives they led
and the example they set for me

———————————

To Albert, my brother and partner for life

A hardcover edition of this book was published by ReganBooks, an imprint of HarperCollins Publishers, in 2001 under the title *Oz Garcia's The Healthy High-Tech Body.*

LOOK AND FEEL FABULOUS FOREVER. Copyright © 2001, 2002 by Oz Garcia. All rights reserved. Printed in the United States of America. No part of this book may be used or reproduced in any manner whatsoever without written permission except in the case of brief quotations embodied in critical articles and reviews. For information address HarperCollins Publishers Inc., 10 East 53rd Street, New York, NY 10022.

HarperCollins books may be purchased for educational, business, or sales promotional use. For information please write: Special Markets Department, HarperCollins Publishers Inc., 10 East 53rd Street, New York, NY 10022.

FIRST PAPERBACK EDITION PUBLISHED 2002.

Designed by Joel Avirom and Jason Snyder
Graphic illustrations by Eli Morgan

The Library of Congress has cataloged the hardcover edition as follows:
Garcia, Oz.
    Oz Garcia's the healthy high-tech body / Oz Garcia, with Sharyn Kolberg.—1st ed.
      p. cm.
    Includes bibliographical references and index.
    ISBN 0-06-039408-0
     1. Medical care—Technological innovations. 2. Medical technology. 3. Technology assessment. I. Kolberg, Sharyn. II. Title.

R855.3.G37 2001
610—dc21
                                                2001031961

ISBN 0-06-098890-8 (pbk.)

02 03 04 05 06 ❖/QW 10 9 8 7 6 5 4 3 2 1

Contents

Acknowledgments

My gratitude and acknowledgments cast a very wide net over people and time. As I've grown and hopefully matured over the years, my office practice and my clients have always forced upon me the request, no, the demand, to stay current and on the forefront of my chosen profession. It's been a long road from where I began on this path twenty-five years ago, when I set out to save the world with my newfound knowledge of vegetarianism. How much better off we would all be if we just grew our own sprouts, ate plenty of brown rice, and juiced all our carrots! My dietary bible then was *Diet for a Small Planet* by Francis Moore Lappe. It has certainly been a long road since then, with a powerful learning curve.

Today I embrace the marvels of science and the great thinkers of our time who continually astonish me with their levels of creative thinking and the great novelty with which they look at all things having to do with human health. I've had the great privilege of meeting some of these individuals as part of writing this book and some have gone on to become friends and colleagues. Their intellectual contributions, which occurred over many long hours of conversation, made this project possible:

Barry Sears, Ph.D.; Ann Louise Gittleman, M.S., C.N.S.; Steven Fowkes; Peter Proctor, M.D.; Steven Levine, Ph.D.; Dave Leonardi, M.D.; Ron Ruden, M.D.; Richard Firshein, O.D.; Harvey Eisenberg, M.D.; Robert Crayhorn, Ph.D.; François de Borne, M.D.; Nicholas Perricone, M.D.; Stephen Bosniak, M.D.; T. S. Wiley; Jim Jamieson, Ph.D.; Jeremy Heaton, M.D.; David Buss; Pamela Peeke, M.D.; Stu Mittleman; Jonathan Bowden, M.S., C.N.S.; Darryl See, M.D.; Deborah Chud, M.D., M.P.H.; Ken Markel, D.D.S.; Loren Pickart, M.D.; Jed Kaminsky, M.D.; Clinique La Prairie; and the Life Extension Foundation.

This book could not have been written without the Internet. It is fitting that a book on all things High Tech and the human body had so much of its knowledge base supported through this instrument of information. I could not have written *Look and Feel Fabulous Forever* without its existence.

My gratitude to: Judith Regan, my publisher and friend. We were out having dinner discussing what my next book project should be. She was multitasking like no one you've ever seen; she whipped out a pen, scribbled out the title of this book on a napkin, took a bite of her dinner, and asked me, "What do you think?" My life has never been the same.

The great Laura Powers, who turned out to be the best right hand I could have wished for on this project. She was a strong project manager and opened doors I never could have without her persistence, charm, and professionalism.

Sharyn Kolberg, who began with me on *The Balance* and has seen me grow into a writer. I relied on her to make sure this book got written properly, and I relied on her to be my "book psychiatrist." She's a great writer with the searing ability to keep objectivity in front of me at all times. I can't wait to do the next book with her.

My brother Albert, the most loyal of all human beings, who has a vision that sustains our dreams and a resolve that makes them come true; we will be partners to the end.

Teddy, our ace in the hole, for having the business sense we need to keep making it all happen.

Crystal, for managing my life and schedule in such a way that time was made, where none existed, to write this book.

Judy Taylor, the best publicist on earth.

Doug Corcoran and Paul Schnee, my editors at Regan Books, for their editing expertise. I am very grateful for the artistic vision of Vanessa Ryan for her book cover design, Eli Morgan for his interior graphic designs, and Alex Krivosheiw for his creative insights.

My special thanks to Martine Friedman and Tom Gregory for their support on this project.

Durk Pearson and Sandy Shaw, for having started so many of us on this path of inquiry with their book, *Life Extension*, written in the early eighties. I still have my original copy, yellowed with notes scribbled on every page. It was a great leap forward for me, not unlike the first time I heard Jimi Hendrix. They simply blew my mind; I hope I do the same for you.

Preface

Aging. It happens to everyone. Even, to my surprise, to me. Not long ago, I found myself at midlife—fifty, to be exact—wondering what I would have to do to enjoy the next twenty, thirty, forty (or more) years that I might live . . . in great condition!

I don't want to live forever. I do want to have eighty to ninety fabulous years.

So far it's been a great life. Lately, though, I've started to experience those things that are universal signals of reaching a certain . . . maturity. I need to wear glasses to read. I can't run at the same pace or with the same stamina I used to. It's become a little more difficult to regulate my weight.

I started to ask myself questions: Is this inevitable? Do I need to worry about things like losing mental clarity, and if, at some point, I might pass some statistical margin that would put my health at risk for any of the so-called diseases of aging? My personal and professional concerns began to move away from managing health to a larger arena—the conservation of faculties, appearance, and physical health and abilities.

Within that arena, several questions arise:

- Are the diseases and maladies of aging inevitable?

- Who out there in this vast world is doing the most innovative work in human improvement and regenerative health and medicine?

- What are the best and most cutting-edge tools available to help us prolong and/or enhance our health and well-being?

Fortunately, I have a privileged vantage point from which to explore and answer these questions, that being my profession for the past twenty years as a successful nutritional consultant in New York City and author of *The Balance,* a bestselling book on the subject of nutritional self-care. I realized my next step was now to develop a broader perspective—an *aerial perspective,* if you will—on the subject matter of **optimal performance** and **successful aging**.

What I discovered was a lot more than I could ever have expected.

This quest turned out to be a yearlong adventure that has taken me physically and digitally around the world. I have spoken to authorities such as researchers, scientists, doctors, pharmacists, paleontologists (yep), experts in fields as new and emerging as *brain performance* and *optimal human sexuality,* as well as to the world's top authorities on *skin elasticity and preservation,* and *hair loss and hair regrowth.*

I found that if I wanted to have this state of exceptional health, I would have to look at the whole picture, not holistically, but *holographically.* I started to realize the relevance of everything: from managing our hormones, to how much sleep we get (yes, we really do need eight hours), to the most advanced diagnostic testing available today to gauge every single level of our health, to the full range of products we can now put to use.

I needed a new, useful understanding of the human biological system, of what the human species could be by taking advantage of the incredible breakthroughs of twenty-first-century science, of how each of us can live those great eighty to ninety years in what I came to call the **Healthy High-Tech Body**.

What Is a Healthy High-Tech Body?

The Healthy High-Tech Body has nothing to do with computerized brains or robotic arms. There are no androids in our immediate future. The Healthy High-Tech Body is not about trying to gain perfection. Having a Healthy High-Tech Body means being able to take advantage of numerous resources available to you in order to obtain and retain the best possible health throughout your lifetime.

Achieving a Healthy High-Tech Body is an ongoing process. It means using the most up-to-date, cutting-edge information in medical, scientific, nutritional, progressive, complementary, holistic, and "health sciences" to:

- perform better at school

- achieve more at your job

- compete better

- feel better

- improve brain function

- maintain a "youthful" appearance

- have the best sex ever

- enable a successful weight loss program

- have a more productive life with your friends and family

- live more high-quality years than you ever thought possible

A Healthy High-Tech Body is a product, and a necessity, of our times.

In order to remain healthy and productive in our later years, we must take advantage now of the best that the world has to offer. Think about it this way: a Healthy

High-Tech Body can help you keep up with the High-Tech world. In order to be highly productive in today's business world, and to preserve the life of your business, you must be well informed about and take advantage of the latest in High-Tech communications systems (like the Internet, networked computers, cell phones, PDAs, etc.). In order to be highly productive and preserve the life of your body, you must be well informed and take advantage of the latest in High-Tech health.

You can start today, at any age, to develop a Healthy High-Tech Body, by taking advantage of the newest inventions, innovations, approaches, products, and techniques to enhance your living experience. With the information in this book, you will be able not only to prolong your life but also to maintain and extend your youthfulness in ways that were not available to previous generations.

A Survivor's Guide

Don't you want to look as great as you can for as long as you can? Wouldn't you like to have an active sexual life into your "senior" years? Don't you want to continue to feel as vital as you did when you were young? Don't you want to cheat heredity and disease and live as long as you can? This book is for those who answered yes to any one of those questions. What you'll find between these pages are the resources, explanations, and information necessary to achieve these ends.

The Healthy High-Tech Body has emerged at a convergent moment in time, when science, technology, medicine, nutrition, pharmaceuticals, and supplementation are all coming together. The good news is that with the information you'll find here you can take advantage of this exciting time in the world of health and make it relevant to your own life. In simple, user-friendly language, you'll discover how to manage and maintain the most important thing in life—your health.

Look and Feel Fabulous Forever is a modern survivor's guide for the changes that are already here and those still ahead of us—in health, in our jobs, in our homes, and in our lives. The result of working with *Look and Feel Fabulous Forever* is that you will gain a new ability to manage your health. You will benefit from the wisdom of over twenty-five leaders and experts in their respective fields, including:

- Dr. Barry Sears, author of *The Zone*, speaking on nutrition

- Dr. Pamela Peeke, author of *Fight Fat After Forty*, speaking about how stress plays a key role in weight gain, hormone fluctuations, and your overall health.

- Dr. Deborah Chud, author of *The Gourmet Prescription*, providing great-tasting, healthy recipes for long life

- Dr. Nicholas Perricone, author of *The Wrinkle Cure*, speaking on how to have everlasting beauty

- Ann Louise Gittleman, author of *Super Nutrition for Women* and *Before the Change*, talking about the importance of understanding hormones

- Dr. Jeremy Heaton, professor at Queen's University in Kingston, Ontario, revealing the latest and future chemistry and drugs for sexuality

- Dr. François de Borne, former head of the Evian Spa in France, speaking on advancements in European cell treatments (you're gonna love this!)

This book puts it all together for you. By following the principles laid out in this book, you, too, can develop your own Healthy High-Tech Body. *You'll be on your way to the best body you've ever had, one that will last you a lifetime.*

Introduction

What is a Healthy High-Tech Body, how you can have one too, and getting the most out of this book

Enhancement ▪ *Rebuilding* ▪ *Repairing* ▪ *Restoration* ▪ *High performance*

Revitalization ▪ *Metabolic efficiency* ▪ *Energy* ▪ *Youthfulness*

Sustained performance ▪ *Power Brain* ▪ *Smart living* ▪ *Amazing sex*

Immune boosting ▪ *Cancer prevention* ▪ *Conserving faculties*

Great hair and skin ▪ *Peace of mind*

And much much more!

We live in an amazing time. Science is bursting at its seams; who knows what incredible breakthroughs tomorrow will bring? What tomorrow will bring is an array of techniques, tools, and surprising new ways for *you* to have the best body possible. That is essentially what *Look and Feel Fabulous Forever* is about. It is a resource that will provide you with the most current information on how to "engineer" great health for yourself. It is important to distinguish at this point the differences in the engineered capabilities offered by breakthroughs in the *biosciences*, at times overwhelming in their imminent promises, and the kind of engineering and results I'm referring to.

We live in times when within a generation or less *genomics, pharmacogenomics, bionic medicine, biotechnologies,* and *nanotechnologies* will literally have transformed how we go about being well and how we define health. We'll no longer be restricted to only what nature can build, but rather by what technologies can custom-design for us. It is a flight from nature, fusing technology with biology that will someday provide treatments for many dreaded genetic diseases and introduce us to virtual iDoctors who will routinely conduct remote heart and brain surgery. An unimaginable amount of genetic research is being conducted at this very minute, the results of which will certainly change the fabric of our society in the not-too-distant future.

This book deals with the practicalities of our lives *now,* with what we can do today so that we can perform to our greatest potential. With so much happening so quickly, it's essential to know what your options are so that you can benefit from superior capabilities at any point in your life, enjoying long-lasting quality of life and deferring infirmity as long as possible, and perhaps looking to make the aging process itself invisible.

In order to achieve these goals I chose the most suitable topics that, in my opinion, when properly exploited, would yield the greatest benefits toward your realizing a higher degree of physical and mental potential.

Achieving a Healthy High-Tech Body is both a product and a necessity of our times. With the latest information and most innovative means available, you can construct a program that will give you an extraordinary edge in today's world. In 1900, life expectancy in industrialized countries was forty-six years; life expectancy today is seventy-seven years. By 2020, one out of every six Americans will be over the age of sixty-five. The odds of your living eighty, ninety, or one hundred years are increasing every day.

The condition you wind up in for the span of your life is in your hands.

Whatever your goal may be in reading this book, from implementing a weight management program that works, to expanding your mental capabilities, to looking great at any age, it's all available by using the information, the tools and techniques of the Healthy High-Tech Body. Just as you have to *retool* in business in order to stay relevant, attractive, and competitive, and to stay in the game, so, too, can you retool your body for the same reasons.

So You Want to Stay in the Game?

Science tells us that our bodies have an amazing ability to heal and repair themselves. This becomes truer when we support this ability with our lifestyles. There is, for instance, a lot of therapeutic power in food. We already know that fruits and vegetables are packed with longevity nutrients. What are longevity nutrients? They're compounds found in food that do everything from reduce the risk of cancer to improve the overall performance of body systems. I'll not only tell you what to eat but what to stay away from and why.

It is a major challenge for each of us to change bad habits, in what we eat, in how (and if) we exercise, in how we take care of ourselves in general. *Look and Feel Fabulous Forever* presents compelling reasons for you to make whatever lifestyle changes are necessary and take advantage of what's out there for you.

The book is divided into five sections or "pillars." Each pillar covers an essential building block of a Healthy High-Tech Body.

Pillar 1: Frontiers

Remember the old saying "The sum is greater than its parts"? Perhaps that statement is truer than ever in these exciting times of bioengineering. Ten years ago cloning was unimaginable; today it is a reality. Dolly the sheep has shown it can be done, for better or worse. For worse, it opens up all kinds of ethical issues (which we will not cover here). For better, it raises incredible possibilities of creating spare parts for humans in need. (You can clone individual organs; they don't have to be harvested from complete individuals.) We're just beginning to understand stem cell therapy and gene therapy treatments. In this chapter you'll learn what they are, how they're currently being used, and how they might be used in the future.

Pillar 2: Supernutrition

The range of health benefits to be derived from how you eat is outlined in this important part of the book, which is called Supernutrition.

This is really the heart of the book; your health depends on it. Chapter 2 is called "The Paleotech Diet" (for reasons you will discover as you read on), and it covers the axioms of a prudent diet plan that will help you restore and maintain much of your health. I have successfully "prescribed" the Paleotech Diet for thousands of clients over twenty years. Some of the results have been:

- improved hormone balances in both men and women

- reduced levels of blood fats such as cholesterol and triglycerides

- reduced blood pressure

- reduced levels of homocysteine, a damaging blood protein implicated in heart disease

- improved immunity and resistance to infection

- improved mood and clarity of mind

- reduced anxiety and diet-induced depression

- reduced inflammatory damage and pain

- increased muscle mass and reduced body fat

- reduced cravings

- improved energy

The Paleotech Diet owes a lot to the science and research pioneered by nutritional authorities such as Drs. Michael and Mary Dan Eades in their seminal books *Protein Power* and *Protein Power Lifeplan;* the rigorous science of Dr. Barry Sears in the Zone franchise of books, especially *The Age-Free Zone*; and the extraordinary work of the evolutionary biologist Loren Cordain at Colorado State University.

The primary benefit of the Paleotech Diet is to give you control over how you feel and look. The full range of benefits that you may experience using this book will become more evident to the extent that you work the Paleotech Diet. *I mean really work it.* Dr. Nicholas Perricone (professor of dermatology at the Yale University School of Medicine), author of *The Wrinkle Cure*, will tell you point-blank that how you eat is crucial to the quality of your skin and appearance. Your skin's luster, tone, and vibrancy are intimately related to the composition of your foods and their potential either to increase wrinkling and inflammation (more on that later) or to slow down the aging process with every morsel you take in.

I've enriched the Paleotech Diet in the chapter called "The Paleotech Gourmet," with terrific recipes from the mind and kitchen of Dr. Deborah Chud, author of *The Gourmet Prescription*. Her sound science regulates the beautiful construction of her meals and will give you a sense of how food that is good for you can be both great tasting and attractively presented.

The Paleotech Diet is extended even further for those of you who are concerned about weight (and who isn't?). In the chapter "High-Tech Secrets of Weight Control," you'll learn about the *complex group of dynamics* that anybody embarking on a weight loss program must address. You'll learn how to jump-start a sluggish metabolism with the "Fat Flush," designed by the nutritional authority and author Ann Louise Gittleman. You'll learn to step off the dieting treadmill and incorporate rational eating practices for maximum fat loss and weight control. And you'll learn how to control your "fat tooth" and your "sweet tooth" as you navigate toward *healthy leanness*.

In order to increase the efficiency of your metabolism even more, chapter 5 covers *nutraceuticals,* the generation of supplements available today that can enhance your health at every level. I'll explain in detail the most important categories of supplements, and the most essential supplements within those categories. You should know that there is a nutraceutical product for almost every concern and compartment of human health. As part of attaining a Healthy High-Tech Body, it's important to understand the potential of everything you consume, from a food to a supplement, and how well it can neutralize what are called "free radicals." Antioxidants stop the damage of very harmful free-radical molecules in our bodies. These nasty molecular terrorists are linked to a warehouse of detrimental effects from illnesses to premature aging and beyond. I'll tell you about powerful antioxidant and supplement therapies that can help protect you against brain disorders such as Alzheimer's disease; supplements that are intended for building muscle, strength, power, and to speed up recovery at any age. Although I'd like this chapter to be definitive and complete, it's neither. It is, rather, my highly refined, focused, and specifically targeted list of the most useful products you can use to optimize your health in the categories I've laid out.

Next, it's vital that we understand that part of the price of living in a High-Tech world is that it is a highly compromised world—overpolluted and extremely toxic. The human body, its tissues and cells (fat cells especially), has the propensity to accumulate and store too much of the metabolic debris left over from what we eat, drink, breathe, and come in physical contact with daily. These offending compounds are called:

carcinogens

neurotoxins

excitotoxins

hormone disruptors

They originate outside our bodies, are in our foods, cleaning agents, paints, all sorts of ubiquitous and common things that "leak" into our skins and stay there. Other factors, like alcohol, tobacco, and prescription and recreational drugs, have extensive documentation as to their toxic damage. We want these toxins out of our bodies because as they accumulate, they produce an unwanted synergy of damage to our brains, our lungs, our livers, and the rest of our bodies. Part of *retooling* is to get these toxins out of our systems. I'll tell you how to accomplish just that in the chapter on Detoxification.

Pillar 3: Life Extension, Life Enhancement

Pillar 3 is concerned with living well longer. That means keeping our bodies—and, above all, our brains—in High-Tech shape no matter how old we are. So we begin with how to have a Power Brain (chapter 7).

> *As our technologies in the developed world continue to improve, muscle strength, coordination, and mechanical skills are becoming less and less important as cognitive skills such as knowledge, intellect, overall mental competence and experience become more important.*
>
> Steven Fowkes, founder of
> The Cognitive Enhancement Research Institute

The Power Brain chapter covers everything you need to know about pumping up your brain muscle to make sure you're prepared to cope, and cope well, throughout your extended lifetime, ranging from basic neuronal maintenance to using the nutraceuticals and drugs that can increase intelligence, improve memory, prevent brain aging, and protect you from "challenging brain disorders." I'll give you winning formulas for a Power Brain so that you can remain mentally strong, protect your brain, and enhance its functions. Although there are no cures currently for the more serious brain disorders, you'll learn about exciting advances in neurological research and how they might affect your future health.

The next two chapters deal with the underlying thread that connects all the sections in the book: the quest to beat aging. There is something called "normal" aging that is being measured as part of the longest-running study being conducted in the United States by the National Institute on Aging's Baltimore Longitudinal Study of Aging (BLSA). This study has supplied us with a "snapshot" of just what aging means today. What you conclude from this study is that the "disease of aging" has a measurable curve to it. You may never be able to not be older, *but* you can do a lot to bring about continual regeneration.

The maximum life span of our species is fixed at about 120 years. Your personal life expectancy is something else altogether. That is determined by any number of factors, including how you live and what happens to you along the way. *Look and Feel Fabulous Forever* is less concerned with your maximum life expectancy and more concerned with *health expectancy*. Research funded by the AARP Andrus Foundation recently concluded that "women can look forward to living free of disability (any condition that significantly impairs independent living, physical functioning, or mental capacity) for about 64 years of their expected life span of 78.8 years; for men, the finding was 60.3 years of an expected life span of 72.6 years." That means that women spend about fifteen years and men about twelve years with at least a moderate disability. The key to having a Healthy High-Tech Body is not how many years you live, but the number of healthy years you can enjoy.

If you have lived a long time but didn't slow the aging process along the way, you have achieved little. The goal of *Look and Feel Fabulous Forever* is to help you maintain *functionality* for as long as possible. As you read this book, you'll be able to customize your own personal quest to beat aging.

Two fascinating High-Tech steps in the quest to beat aging are the use of *cell therapy* and *human growth hormone therapy*. I visited Clinique La Prairie in Switzerland, one of the world's foremost anti-aging institutions and the place where cell therapy was born. I also visited the premier American anti-aging clinic, Cenegenics, in Las Vegas. In addition, I had the privilege of chatting up Dr. François de Borne, former head of the Evian anti-aging clinic in France. There is plenty of controversy over these treatments. You can take them or leave them, but you have to know about them. Cell treatments and human growth hormone therapy are currently on the front line of clinical anti-aging protocols, and already draw thousands of adherents. You may want to consider these powerful tools, as I did, for their life-enhancing properties.

Before you can work on extending your current life and health expectancy, however, you have to have the right information about your current state of health. In chapter 10 you'll discover the latest breakthroughs in diagnostics and functional analysis. These are new ways of finding out what is wrong with you—and what is right. There are new tests available to fully assess your metabolic functions, your gastrointestinal tract, your hormones, your nutritional and immune status.

Being well informed through functional analysis is a key element that defines a more proactive form of healthcare, supporting what is being called Functional Medicine, an approach that is geared toward keeping you healthy rather than treating you after you're already sick.

Pillar 4: The Body Beautiful

The visible signs of aging often appear well before we're ready for them. That's because aging is a form of *organic rusting* that seeps into every part of the body. It is the result of two processes moving relentlessly together to produce everything from wrinkling and age spots to nail discoloration. Controlling these two processes, *oxidation* and *glycation*, are passageways to a beautiful body. Chapter 11, "Looking Good Longer," explains the concept of "cosmeceuticals," which will help restore a great complexion (and add to your overall good health). I'll also let you in on several nonsurgical advancements to keep the premature aging of your skin in check.

You'll also learn about another insight into what makes us age: gum disease. It turns out that gingivitis and periodontal disease cause problems in both the immune and arterial systems. For instance, studies have shown that men under the age of fifty who have advanced periodontal disease are 2.6 times more likely to die prematurely and 3 times more likely to die from heart disease than men who have healthy teeth and gums. You'll also find what the world of dentistry has got in store for you to help you keep your teeth, and keep them healthy, as long as you live.

Then, of course, there's the subject of hair. In chapter 12 you'll find out how to keep the hair you have and how to stop what you've got left from falling out. We may not have the cure for balding yet, but we've got many more options than we had just five years ago.

The final chapter in this pillar is all about keeping limber. It goes beyond the exercise discussed in Pillar 2, into high-level fitness. I used to run marathons and work out seven days a week. Throughout my twenties and into my early forties I kept up this grueling pace. And then I started getting *injured*!

I had to rethink the whole nature of how I was to stay fit and keep my muscle mass and body fat levels within acceptable ranges. I had to find an exercise routine that was appropriate to my needs—but one that wouldn't kill me in the process. I began to study the *kind* of exercise we need as we age, and I started to realize that there was more to life (and health) than aerobics. A key biological marker of aging is the loss of muscle mass and strength. Estimates are that we lose 25 to 30 percent of our muscle mass and strength by age sixty-five. That's six pounds of muscle mass lost with each passing decade. I'll share with you the current thinking on what kind of exercise is best to keep an aging body at peak performance levels.

I'll also share the most up-to-the minute findings on arthritis—what you can do to help prevent it from happening, and how you can deal with it if it does. Keeping limber, keeping your joints properly lubricated, and maintaining "plasticity" in your body tissues are all things you can begin doing now to ensure that you stay mobile as you age (which comes in handy in order to enjoy the next pillar even more!).

Pillar 5: Sexuality

There's only one chapter in this pillar. It's about sex. Let's be frank: at fifty years of age, I really wanted to know, *for myself,* how to keep it "going" for the next fifty years. There are many things we still don't understand about sex and sexuality. There are some solutions that work better than others. It's a complex, sometimes confusing topic. This chapter will present you with what science currently knows and what High-Tech doctors and pharmacologists are doing to help create a healthier sexuality that does not have to diminish with age. In addition, you'll find the latest information on PMS and menopause for women and andropause (the male equivalent) for men, and discover how to cooperate with nature as your body begins to shift its gears. *Welcome to the new sexual potency.*

Appendix A: Some Cool Stuff

Scientists are studying many other things besides the human body to engineer a better future. There's a lot of cool stuff out there. For instance, there's a device that controls microbe growth. (Howard Hughes would've loved this device.) This chapter contains a wide variety of the best, most innovative products from some very cool companies that will make your life easier, safer, and healthier.

Appendix B: The Five Pillars Updated

Time marches on, and so does High-Tech science. Since this book was first published there have been many new developments in each of the five pillars. Discover how the frontiers are expanding with research into human therapeutic cloning. Learn how scientists are working to win the war against obesity, and what new nutraceuticals you should add to your High-Tech arsenal. Check out the amazing advancements in European cell treatments, using stem cells still not approved for use in the United States. And be introduced to Mésothérapie, a revolutionary European therapy used to treat skin ailments such as cellulite, sagging, and stretch marks. Finally, find out about the most advanced natural hormone treatments available by prescription.

So . . .

It's taken many millions of years for us to move through the evolutionary struggle that produced *Homo sapiens*. Over all those years, we've developed science and technology to help us survive and thrive and live in a modern world. In other ways, however, science and technology have led us astray, into an overfed, overprocessed, toxic world. How we choose to live in *this* High-Tech world may determine the future of our species. You can use the remarkable information within this book to have a better body, a better environment, a better you. And have fun along the way. Welcome to *Look and Feel Fabulous Forever*.

Pillar 1
Frontiers

Come in to the "house of tomorrow"—or in this case, the body of
tomorrow. We could never have imagined in the middle of the twentieth century
the kinds of scientific achievements that have been developed at the beginning of
the twenty-first. Maybe an old *Twilight Zone* episode comes to mind, one in which
people are constructed of old spare parts, where the difference between humans
and machines is hardly detectable.

We're not there yet, but we're getting close. The Human Genome Project is giving us an understanding of the human mechanism we have never seen before.
We're just beginning to get some idea of what applications this new understanding
will bring.

But just to give you a glimpse, "Bioengineering" will explain what's going on
now and what's coming up in the fields of stem cell and gene therapies. How we
may be able to clone organs for transplants so that one person doesn't have to die
to save another's life. How doctors may be able to study our genes and prescribe
custom-designed medications and treatments based on our individual genetic
makeup. How tiny cameras can travel through our bodies and help doctors see how
we're doing from the inside out. How operations can be performed in one room by
a doctor sitting in another room thousands of miles away.

It is the stuff of science fiction fast becoming science fact.

1 Bioengineering

Moving medicine forward

In the time it will take you to read this book, there may have been hundreds of medical discoveries that bring us closer to a Healthy High-Tech Body than ever before. New discoveries in medicine are moving at an almost unimaginable rate. In a perfect marriage of biology and technology, scientists are using knowledge from the fields of medicine and engineering to help us all live longer, and live better.

We live in a world of paradox. We still cannot cure the common cold (although we're getting close), but we can successfully exchange failing organs for ones that bring us back to life. We can't solve the problem of the epidemic of obesity, but we have broken the entire human genetic code—not that we even know what that really means for the future of mankind. We know—almost—how to build babies in petri dishes; we just don't know if it's right to do so.

The science of health is now spread out in many directions, with research projects exploring many fronts, some of which are described below. This chapter is not about predictions of where medicine might go in the future, but rather about possibilities. Some of the techniques and inventions presented are just around the corner from reality; others are years away. Some will become common practice in our lifetime; some will be beneficial not to us, but to our grandchildren. It's impossible to say right now what the next big breakthrough will be. However, the fields that are receiving the most attention here at the beginning of the twenty-first century include the following:

- telemedicine

- robotic surgery

- nanotechnology

- home-based diagnostics tools

- transplants

- stem cell therapy

- gene therapy

Telemedicine: Seeing the Doctor Without "Seeing" the Doctor

In 1999, Dr. Jerri Nielsen went to the South Pole as part of a research team. She was prepared for the cold and the hardships of such an adventure; she was not prepared for cancer. Dr. Nielsen was the only medical doctor in her group. As soon as she found a lump in her breast, she knew she was in for trouble. Because of the winter weather conditions, she could not leave the Pole, nor could anyone fly in to help her. How could she even diagnose herself, no less treat her own disease?

The only possible way to save her life was through the use of telemedicine. Because she was able to communicate, via computer, with doctors thousands of miles away, Dr. Nielsen and her colleagues were able to save her life. Had this technology not existed, the doctor would surely have perished long before she could get out of that frozen land.

Simply put, telemedicine is the use of telecommunications to provide medical information and services. This technology enables doctors to communicate with specialists at long distances, as well as allowing patients to communicate with their doctors. There are two basic types of technology that are currently being used in this field:

1. Store and forward This is when a digital image is stored at one location and then sent to another. This method is used in teleradiology, when X rays, CT scans, or MRI results are sent from one medical center to another or from a medical center to an individual doctor. Some radiologists even have the appropriate computer technology installed at home so that they can have images sent to them directly for diagnosis. This technology is also used in the field of telepathology, where images of pathological slides are sent from one location to another for diagnosis (which is how Dr. Nielsen's tumor was biopsied).

2. Two-way interactive television This technology is used when a "live" consultation is necessary. Dr. Nielsen used this technology so that doctors could guide her through her cancer treatment. You don't have to be at the South Pole to have need for this kind of technology. It's extremely useful for anyone in a rural area, far from an urban health center or specialist. There are programs that currently use desktop videoconferencing systems. You can even attach peripheral devices, such as a stethoscope, to make examination and diagnosis easier.

There are many examples of how this technology is currently being used to save lives worldwide. In Canada, a program called SmartLabrador was set up to include telemedicine for all Labrador nursing stations and health centers. In Greenland, hospitals and towns in the country's twenty largest settlements will be linked by telemedical technology by the year 2002, making telemedicine available to over 50 percent of the population. The United Nations is sponsoring a telemedicine program that will allow children's hospitals around the world to consult with American hospitals and specialists to help children who are catastrophically ill.

Closer to home, some cities in the United States are using telemedicine to allow school nurses to consult with physicians, and telemedicine is being used in correctional facilities so that prisoners do not have to be transported to health centers.

The city of Baltimore, Maryland, is conducting a study using telemedicine to link patients in ambulances to a neurologist at the University of Maryland Medical Center to help stroke patients get the treatment they need as soon as possible. And the Visiting Nurse Associations of America is using a device that is individually programmed by a physician and placed in a patient's home to collect real-time vital data. When the patient gets up in the morning, he or she is voice-prompted to check vital signs such as heart rate, blood pressure, and lung function. The information is then sent to a central station for evaluation. If there is a problem, both patient and doctor will know it immediately.

In Japan, Mitsushita Electric is testing a suitcase-size telemedical box to be kept in the home. It contains a thermometer, a glucose meter, a miniature electrocardiogram machine, and a video camera so that patients can perform tests on themselves, send the data to their doctors, and then have a face-to-face conference if necessary.

Robotic Surgery: Medicine's Longest Reach

The concept of telemedicine began with no more than two doctors consulting over long-distance phone lines. Now it is possible not only for doctors (and patients) to consult over previously inconceivable distances, but also for doctors to participate actively in surgery—without touching a patient—from across the room or from thousands of miles away.

Not long ago, a patient in Baltimore had a damaged nerve cut and cauterized by a doctor in Chicago. A woman in Virginia had her gallbladder removed by two steel "arms" while her doctor sat a few feet away at a computer console. And the year 2000 saw the first American coronary bypass surgery performed by a robot called da Vinci.

Robotic surgery is not a vision for the future. It is technology that is slowly being introduced to hospital operating rooms across the country, for a limited number of operations. The Food and Drug Administration has to approve each new use. But scientists estimate that eventually robotic surgery will be used in more than four million medical procedures each year in the United States alone.

Here's an example of how robotic surgery works. You need your gallbladder removed. You are prepped and readied as for any standard operation. The doctor sits at a computer console, which can be located anywhere in the room, or in the hospital, a different hospital, a different state, or a different country. Three tiny incisions are made into your abdomen, and three stainless steel rods are inserted. One of these rods is equipped with a camera. The other two are fitted with surgical instruments that are able to dissect and suture the tissue of the damaged organ (in this case, the gallbladder). At the console, the doctor views on a video screen the images being relayed by the camera that's inside your body. He then uses joystick-like controls, located beneath the video screen, to manipulate the surgical instruments.

There are many advantages to this kind of robotic or telesurgery. It usually takes almost a dozen people to perform even a simple surgical operation. Robotics can reduce that number greatly. It also can take many hours to perform surgery, with the doctor having to stand over the patient the whole time. Now he or she can sit at a console while the robotic arms do the hard work. The robot doesn't suffer from fatigue, which is when many surgeons' hands begin to shake and mistakes and accidents occur.

The greatest advantage, however, is to recovery time. Traditional heart bypass surgery, for instance, requires that a patient's chest be "cracked" open with a one-foot-long incision. Using robotic surgery, it is possible to operate on the heart by making three small incisions in the chest, each only about one centimeter in diameter. Because of these much smaller incisions, patients experience less bleeding and a lot less pain, which means they experience a much shorter recovery time.

At this exciting time in medicine, there are unlimited possibilities for this technology. It is currently being studied by NASA for use with astronauts. Fortunately, there has never been a serious medical emergency in space. But what if there was? Using robotic technology, doctors could conceivably use telemanipulation to direct surgery over millions of miles so that no astronaut need ever be "lost in space." And, scary as the thought may be, the twenty-first century just might see the advent of robotics, powered by artificial intelligence, able to diagnose, analyze, and operate on human abnormalities with no human help at all.

Nanotechnology: Medicine's Smallest Reach

Now that we have seen large machines that operate through tiny incisions, what's next? Robots the size of a hyphen might just be next. A company in Israel has already invented a pill-size video camera that travels through the digestive tract, transmitting pictures as it goes. The device is made of a camera and a light source, radio transmitters, and batteries, all housed within a sealed capsule slightly more than an inch long and less than half an inch wide. It is intended to replace the current endoscopic procedure for examining the small intestine. Now an examination of the full intestine requires that tubes be inserted into a sedated patient's body. The camera-in-a-pill is simply swallowed, and the patient goes about his or her daily routine for the next twenty-four to forty-eight hours. The camera continues to transmit pictures and sends out signals so that the doctor knows where in the digestive tract a particular image was taken. Although this device has already been tested and shown to work in human subjects, the goal of the company is eventually to design a device that will be able to repair problems as well as view them.

The science that makes this tiny technology possible is called nanotechnology. The word *nano* comes from the Greek word for dwarf, but it has since come to mean "a billionth." The goal is to build incredibly small machines—smaller than the diameter of a human hair—that will be able to travel through veins, arteries, and even capillaries. They will be designed to sense viruses or cancers and attack enemy cells. They would then be able to build healthy cells right where the body needs them.

Dr. Michio Kaku, a professor at the City University of New York and author of the book *Visions*, told MSNBC, "Nanotechnology may give us the power of a god to be able to conceive objects and then create them almost like magic, to be able to manipulate atom for atom any object around us, but it also means we have to have the wisdom to go with it." That wisdom is leading some scientists toward inventing molecule-sized motors (a hundred thousand would fit on the head of a pin) that might someday be used to move one single cell from one point in the body to another.

Great Gadgets: Problem Detectors

Much of the science of tomorrow is focusing on even more ways to prevent disease from occurring, or at least catching it early, before it can do great damage. The focus is also on devising ways to make medicine more personalized and individualized, so that medicine will eventually be less "one cure fits all" and more "this is what *your* body needs."

This is the philosophy of researchers like Philippe Fauchet, chair of the electrical and computer engineering department of the University of Rochester. He told *Popular Science* magazine in July 2000 that the current system of waiting until you get sick, then diagnosing what you have, then sending you for "multi-million-dollar technology such as MRI machines" is "a pretty inefficient use of resources because it waits until the patient sees there's something wrong. That can be very late in the development of a disease."

That's why places like the University of Rochester and MIT (and research labs around the world) are developing High-Tech products that can be used in the home to scan various body parts and functions and compare them to your established norm. We already have scales that tell us our body fat percentage as well as our weight, and home-based glucose, heart rate, and blood pressure monitors. So what's next? Here are some possibilities:

Memory glasses Day-Timers and Palm Pilots could go the way of the horse-drawn buggy once these glasses are perfected. They would work like a human appointment book, delivering reminders for meetings, taking pills, making phone calls, etc. They could also contain a miniature camera, programmed to recognize certain visual images. They could tell you, for instance, "The person standing in front of you is your nephew Jake."

Mole patrol A small digital camera mounted in your shower could take timed photos (every one or two months) and compare the moles on your body to the photos it took the month before. It would send out a warning if it detected any changes in the color, shape, or size of the moles.

The tell-all toothbrush Researchers are working on a toothbrush that would contain sensors to check your breath and/or your saliva, analyze your proteins, and let you know if you have any of the telltale markers for an imminent heart attack. If the sensors detected levels that differed from your norm, they would send out a warning signal letting you know you need an immediate checkup.

The bed rest bed test Tiny sensors and ultra-thin fiber-optic cables could be built into your mattress to monitor sleep patterns and vital signs, such as blood pressure and heart rate. Your bed could let you know if you have sleep apnea or even measure your snoring decibel.

Transplants:
The Science of Spare Parts

The day when nanorobots can repair damaged organs and cells is still well in the future. One area of science that is making great strides today is organ transplants.

Unfortunately, those strides are not quick enough for the more than 75,400 men, women, and children on the national organ transplant waiting list. More than 48,000 are waiting for kidneys, 17,000 for livers, 4,000 for hearts, and 3,700 for lungs (statistics as of March 24, 2001, by the United Network for Organ Sharing, which manages the nationwide transplant network). Of those 75,000-plus people waiting, less than one-third will get the transplants they need.

The good news is that we have come a long way since 1954, when the first successful kidney transplant, from one twin to another, was completed, and from 1967, when the first liver and heart transplants were completed. Those first operations were successful, but the patients did not survive very long. New studies have shown that, because of improved surgical techniques, greater success at keeping grafted organs healthy, and better antirejection drugs, transplant patients are living much longer than they did ten years ago.

Scientists are constantly trying to perfect the transplant process and are making progress every year. In 1999, the first hand transplant in the United States was performed on a man who had lost his hand in an accident eleven years previously.

Every half hour, someone in the world receives an organ transplant; however, every two hours and twenty-four minutes someone dies waiting for an organ to save his or her life. You can become an organ donor by downloading an organ donation card from www.shareyourlife.org or by calling 888-355-SHARE.

The man does not have full use of the new hand, but he can hold a glass of water, tie his shoes, and feel heat, cold, and pain. Great strides have also been made in an altogether different area of the body—the intestines. This is vital for both children and adults who have lost intestinal function due to disease, injury, or abnormalities at birth. Without transplants, most of these people can survive only through intravenous feeding. One advantage of being able to transplant intestines is that, although children need donors of their own height and weight, the intestine, like the liver, has the ability to regenerate and will grow as the child does. In fact, liver transplants are now being done from living donors. Because the liver can regenerate itself, surgeons can cut out a large chunk of a live donor's liver and transplant it into another adult.

Of course, most transplants can only take place when appropriate donors are found. Right now, those donors are cadavers. But even though millions of people die every year, only about 2 percent are potential organ donors. So scientists are looking for ways to replace damaged organs without having to wait for people to die. With that in mind, there are two main areas of research going on: xenotransplants and bioartificial organs.

Xenotransplants A xenotransplant is a transplant between two different species. Perhaps the most well-known xenotransplant recipient was "Baby Faye," who was born with a malformed heart and survived for twenty days in 1984 with a baboon heart. Extensive research into xenotransplantation is now going on around the world, and much of it is being conducted on pigs. That is because a pig's internal organs are fairly similar to those of a human. And pigs can be bred for the sole purpose of supplying organs to humans who need them. The problem with using pig organs, of course, is that the human immune system is built to reject foreign tissue. When an animal's (or even another human being's) organ is placed in a body, that body will send antibodies to kill the foreign cells. That's why transplant patients have to take antirejection drugs for the rest of their lives. The rejection of another species' tissues is even more violent than the rejection of human tissue. So scientists are experimenting by breeding genetically altered animals, adding human genes to the pigs. The hope is not that humans will be able to live with pig organs forever, but that they will be able to tolerate them in order to stay alive long enough to receive a human organ.

There are great concerns in transplanting animal organs into humans, and many countries have imposed moratoriums on such transplants until more research is done. The greatest fear is that along with the organs, we may be transplanting viruses that are dangerous—if not fatal—to humans. It may be that animal transplants could unleash another AIDS epidemic. That disease apparently originated in monkeys and was somehow transmitted to humans; scientists fear that an unknown virus equally harmful to man could be lurking in pigs.

Bioartifical organs One possible solution to the problems listed above is the bioartificial organ, which is a combination of live cells and mechanical devices. David Pescovitz, writing for *Scientific American,* described the process: "The strategy thus far is to take organ cells from humans or pigs, grow them in a culture medium, then load them into a bioreactor—a box or tube in which they are kept alive with oxygen and nutrients. The bioreactor is inserted into a larger machine outside the body. A patient's blood is diverted via tubes through the bioreactor, where it is cleansed—similar to the setup of today's kidney dialysis machines."

Devices are now in use or in development to aid damaged kidneys and livers. The bioartificial liver, for instance, is used in patients who are suffering from acute liver failure, a condition that progresses rapidly from jaundice to coma. It is estimated that up to 80 percent of these patients will die without a liver transplant—and many of them pass away before a viable organ can be found. There is also a device that

Research is now under way using genetically engineered mice that can make antibodies just like the ones produced by the human body. So far, two U.S. firms have patented strains of genetically modified mice that make human antibodies when injected with an antigen (a disease-causing organism or substance). Hybridized antibodies—made by slicing mouse-made antibodies into human antibodies—are already in use in several drugs, including Herceptin, which inhibits the growth of many cancer cells. However, because these cells are not totally human, they can cause side effects, including nausea, extreme allergic reactions, and even heart failure. Scientists hope that the antibodies produced by genetically engineered mice will not cause these kinds of side effects and can then be used to treat almost any kind of disease, from infections to cancer.

uses insulin-producing tissue from pigs to supply diabetic patients with the insulin they need. These devices, too, are intended to serve as stopgap measures until appropriate human organs can be transplanted.

Stem Cell Therapy: Living Longer with Replacement Parts

The logical extension of all this research into transplantation is, of course, finding ways to manufacture whole new organs from "scratch" so that no one would have to depend on another person's death to give them life. These organs could be made in one of two ways. In the first, a patient's failing organ would be injected with a particular molecule, such as a growth factor. These molecules would cause the patient's own cells to migrate to that organ and regenerate tissue. In the second case, cells that have been previously harvested (from the patient or from a donor) are placed into a sort of polymer mold, designed to dissolve in the body. The mold is then placed into the body, where the cells replicate and form new tissue as the polymers dissolve. In the end, you're left with a new organ.

This procedure is already being implemented, either in practice or in clinical trial, by several hospitals using fabricated skin, cartilage, bone, ligaments, and tendons. Research is also under way to use tissue from the legs or buttocks to grow new breast tissue for women who have had lumpectomies or mastectomies.

Replacing failing body parts is the ultimate goal of regenerative medicine: not just to fix up a sick body, but to supplant old and damaged tissues with young, healthy ones. As Dr. William Haseltine, chief executive of Human Genome Sciences, told Nicholas Wade of the *New York Times* (November 7, 2000): "When we know, in effect, what our cells know, health care will be revolutionized, giving birth to regenerative medicine—ultimately including the prolongation of life by regenerating our aging bodies with younger cells."

But where do we get these "younger cells"? The answer to that question is stem cells. In its "Stem Cells: A Primer," the National Institutes of Health includes this definition:

> [Stem cells] are best described in the context of normal human development. Human development begins when a sperm fertilizes an egg and creates a single cell that has the potential to form an entire organism. . . . Approximately four days after fertilization and after several cycles of cell division, these . . . cells begin to specialize, forming a hollow sphere of cells, called a blastocyst. The blastocyst has an outer layer of cells and inside the hollow sphere, there is a cluster of cells called the inner cell mass. . . . The outer layer will go on to form the placenta and other supporting tissues needed for fetal development in the uterus. The inner cell mass cells will go on to form virtually all of the tissues in the human body.

These inner mass cells, or stem cells, are pluripotent, which means they can give rise to many different types of cells. There are essentially two types of stem cells:

Embryonic stem cells These are derived from the earliest development stages of the embryo (the blastocyst). They have an unlimited ability to divide, and they have the capability to turn into any and all cell types and tissues in the body. There are ethical issues beyond the scope of this book involved in using these cells, so scientists are looking for alternatives. There is even research being done into making human embryonic stem cells by fusing adult human cells with a cow's egg. These results have yet to be tested.

Adult stem cells Once embryonic cells form the body, the stem cells basically disappear, leaving only a relatively few descendants to keep around for repairing the body when needed. These descendants are called adult stem cells. Adult stem cells usually replenish themselves within their own type: neural stem cells make brain cells; bone marrow cells make red and white blood cells. But as Nicholas Wade noted in his *New York Times* article, "In laboratory experiments . . . several types of adult stem cells seem to be able to take on other types' roles; perhaps, with the right signals, an adult stem cell will repair any tissue, not just its own." Recent studies seem to bear this out. Experiments in mice seem to show that neural stem cells placed into the bone marrow produce brain cells.

There are several drawbacks in using adult stem cells. Adult stem cells have not been identified for all tissue types. Adult stem cells seem to decrease with age and are difficult to isolate and purify. And if you wanted to use stem cells from a patient's own body, you would first have to harvest them from the patient, then grow them in a culture in sufficient numbers required for the treatment. For many people who are seriously ill, this process would simply take too long.

Despite the drawbacks of both kinds of stem cells, they both contain enormous promise and may prove to revolutionize the way we practice medicine. In March 2001, for instance, two studies involving adult stem cells offered hope for their eventual use in repairing damaged hearts. In a study led by the National Human Genome Research Institute, researchers harvested bone marrow stem cells from male mice. Heart attacks were induced in several female mice, and the harvested stem cells were injected into the heart muscle next to the damaged tissue. Within two weeks, the stem cells began to multiply and transform themselves into heart muscle cells and migrated to the damaged area. They also began producing cells that organized themselves into new blood vessels.

A second study, conducted at the Columbia University College of Physicians and Surgeons, injected a special kind of stem cell from human bone marrow, called an angioblast, into rats after a heart attack. The cells migrated to the damaged heart tissue and spurred the formation of new blood vessels. Similar studies are being conducted on pigs' hearts. It is very possible that the same technique can be used to save human hearts.

Gene Therapy:
Curing Disease Before It Starts

Stem cell therapy concentrates on using existing cells to create new ones in order to repair some damaged body part. There is another branch of High-Tech scientific research that is studying ways to prevent the lethal and disabling diseases we inherit through our genes. Genes are what make us who we are: they determine everything from height to hair color. Unfortunately, they can also sometimes lead to the development of disease.

The object of gene therapy is to allow normal genes to be inserted into a patient's cells to replace or counteract defective or missing genes. There are two types of gene therapy. **Somatic gene therapy** corrects a problem in a particular patient, but these corrections are not inherited by the next generation. This is the type of therapy that is being researched today. The second type is called **germline (egg or sperm) gene therapy**, and this involves modification of cells that will be passed on to the next generation. Due to technical and ethical reasons, this type of therapy is not currently being studied.

In June 2000, scientists from the Human Genome Project and the private company Celera announced that they had completed a draft of the map to the human genetic code. Their goal was to identify all human genes and map the genes' locations on chromosomes. The completed map should allow scientists to identify specific genes that lead to specific diseases. The most immediate application of that will be in diagnostics. As each "disease gene" is identified, a new test will appear to determine your own hereditary risk for that disease.

Genetic Testing

Some types of genetic screening already exist, for breast cancer and Huntington's disease, among others. Most tests can tell you if you are predisposed to the disease, not whether you will actually get it. There are many diseases that are influenced by environment and behavior, so that even if you are predisposed to diabetes, for example, you may be able to avoid it by your dietary and lifestyle choices. Other diseases can be monitored and caught early enough to be arrested or cured. Right now, most genetic tests available are for relatively rare diseases for which an individual might be at risk. For instance, if you have a family history of Huntington's disease, you can get tested and find out with a high degree of certainty if the disease is already present or if there is a good chance that it will develop.

We have not yet reached the stage (and it is probably a long way off) where you get a complete analysis of your entire genome to see what may or may not be there.

Pharmacogenomics

Another important result of gene identification could be to tell you if your genes predispose you to positive or negative reactions to particular drugs. Right now, scientists develop one drug that is meant to help millions of people in the same way. However, gene research is telling us that genetic differences influence how we absorb, break down, and respond to various drugs. An article in the July 2000 issue of *Scientific American* stated that "until now, the genome generators have focused on the similarities among us all. Scientists think that 99.9 percent of your genes perfectly match those of the person sitting beside you. But the remaining 0.1 percent of your genes vary—and it is these variations that most interest drug companies."

What that means is that sometime in the future, when you go to your pharmacist to get your medication, it will be based on your individual genetic profile. The person standing behind you, with the same illness, will get a different version of the same medication, making for precise, customized treatment.

Creating the Perfect Specimen

There may be nothing that intrigues humans more than the ability to make perfect replicas of themselves. To some this is the road that gene therapy should follow. Everyone knows about Dolly, the cloned sheep created in Scotland in 1997. Since then, many other cloned animals have been created. But is it really possible to make "designer babies"? Perhaps. Perhaps not. But scientists may have taken the first steps, however small. In early 2001, scientists created the first genetically modified primate, a rhesus monkey named ANDi, whose name stands for "inserted DNA" backward. An extra marker gene was introduced to the unfertilized egg that was used to create him. This was the first time that scientists were able to study a gene-modified primate, the animal that is closest to human in makeup. The hope is that it will allow scientists to study diseases that are too difficult to study in rodents, the animals usually used in such studies.

However, experts warn that we are not quite ready to produce people inserted with "just the right" genes. As Arthur Caplan, director of the Center for Bioethics at the University of Pennsylvania in Philadelphia, told MSNBC, the research team that created ANDi "chose a benign gene that naturally glows when it is just sitting there. They didn't choose a gene that actually did anything. . . . That's a long way from creating a 7-foot, redheaded, basketball-playing, superstar model. To do that, you have to use genes that work and get them to go where they need to go. . . . Scientists can't control where the inserted gene enters the genome, so there is no telling what could happen if it ended up in the wrong place."

To many people, cloning seems to be just around the corner. But the reality is that most animal clones die during embryonic development. Some are stillborn, showing terrible abnormalities. And the surrogate mothers that carry clone embryos often suffer difficult pregnancies and risky miscarriages.

Here, at the beginning of the twenty-first century, there is no telling what the future of medical science holds. The only thing we can predict is that the discoveries that come tomorrow will be more amazing than anything we can imagine today.

Pillar 2

Supernutrition

Now that we've looked at what the future may hold, it's time to concentrate on building a Healthy High-Tech Body today. If you want to "live long and prosper," this is where you start. If you want the best body that science (and nature) can offer, look first to food. You don't have to be a scientist to know that food is the fuel on which the human machine runs. What scientists are now helping us understand is the chemical aspect of food and how those chemicals interact with the chemicals in our body's systems.

We all understand the concept of drug interactions. We read labels and heed warnings that caution us against taking certain types of drugs with certain other types of drugs. We also know that many drugs are extremely dangerous when taken with alcohol. What we don't know, and what *The Healthy High-Tech Body* will tell you, is that food is a powerful drug as well, and—if we want to live long, healthy lives—we must be very careful about how we mix it with the chemical agents that naturally reside within our bodies.

The kinds of foods we eat have a direct, chemical-based effect on us from the first bite we take in the morning to the last snack before bedtime. Food modifies our hormones. It can improve or impair our metabolism. It can increase or decrease our energy levels. It can strengthen or weaken our concentration and brain performance. And scientists now know that there is a direct connection between food—specifically the nutrients derived from food—and a healthy or compromised immune system.

It's clear from the outset that for you to reap the advantages of the scientific breakthroughs in all the other pillars in this book, you've got to address your diet first.

What You'll Find Here

This Supernutrition pillar is the linchpin of the Healthy High-Tech Body. Chapter 2, "The Paleotech Diet," will teach you how to construct a way of eating that's appropriate for you, that will help you enjoy extraordinarily good health, and will possibly even extend your life. You'll learn how to use food therapeutically to improve your immune system and reduce your risk of cancer and cardiovascular disease. You'll not only discover a whole new way of eating based on human paleological history, you'll also find out what's wrong with the way we eat in the modern world, and how it may be killing you and those you love.

In chapter 3, you'll find not only what to eat but also delicious ways to prepare it in gourmet recipes developed especially for the High-Tech Body.

Chapter 4, "High-Tech Secrets of Weight Control," will reveal why we're becoming an obese nation. You'll learn why we store fat where we store it and what makes you fat and what doesn't. You'll learn about all the behaviors that affect your weight—not just your eating habits but your exercise and your sleep habits. You'll find out why conventional diets don't work, no matter how much willpower you apply, and what science has to say about some of the current fads that make "overnight weight loss" claims. By following the guidelines in this chapter (and the rest of this book), you'll learn the healthiest and most effective ways to use food to increase metabolism, burn fat, and lose weight.

Chapter 5, "High-Tech Neutraceuticals," explores some of the most progressive supplements on the market today to burn fat, to improve your energy, to reduce your risk of illness, and to improve how your brain performs. You'll discover which vitamins, minerals, essential fats, amino acids, and herbs are safe and effective for you to use. You'll find out about some European products that are now available and how you can obtain them. You won't find out about every supplement out there—this is not an exhaustive list—but you will learn about which ones are going to make the biggest difference in achieving your goals for a Healthy High-Tech Body.

The final chapter in this pillar concerns detoxification. In our modern world, not only our food is making us sick, but there are toxins that appear in what we eat, what we drink, and what we breathe. Hundreds, if not thousands, of toxic compounds are embedded in many foods and products we use. Medical drugs also often leave behind a toxic residue that stays in the body long after they're consumed. Over a lifetime, you accumulate huge amounts of neurotoxins, excitotoxins, and hormone disrupters. These are compounds and chemicals that appear in our food and our water supplies that have the nasty habit of winding up in our bodies, possibly affecting us throughout our lives.

If you want to have a High-Tech Body, if you want to have vibrant health, it will be essential also to understand what it means to cleanse and detoxify your body. You'll find out how detoxification can be used to revitalize you in a way that you have not felt in years. Chapter 6 will teach you how to incorporate a simple detoxifying and cleansing program that will complement and reinforce your eating and supplementation programs, and have the maximum impact on your health and well-being.

Pursuing the Healthy High-Tech Body is not just a matter of living longer. It's living longer healthier, retaining and even improving your quality of life as you age. The next five chapters will get you started on a fantastic journey to vibrant health, supernutrition, and the Healthy High-Tech Body.

2 The Paleotech Diet

Looking to the future
with an eye to the past

The Big Picture

If you want to peer into the High-Tech future of the human race, you have to look to its most low-tech past. The most important fact to keep in mind is that human beings are animals—primates, to be exact. As such, we have certain fundamental requirements that must be met to ensure our survival. We must have air to breathe. We must have water to drink. And we must have food to eat.

The quality of the air we breathe and the water we drink may have declined somewhat over the thousands of years humans have existed; however, it remains substantially the same as it was forty thousand years ago. It still satisfies our genetic requirements.

The same cannot necessarily be said about food.

In fact, food has a long and extraordinary history. In order to achieve the goals of the Healthy High-Tech Body, we're going to review some of it, because *your relationship to food and its impact on your health means everything*. The modern American diet has undergone a transformation of such magnitude as to constitute a new type of nourishment—if you can call it that—that we'll call *nufood*.

Our changing lifestyles and our never-ending quest for convenience have radically redefined what we eat and how we eat it. Nufood barely satisfies our genetic requirements. It does not fulfill food's primary functions of providing the mortar for building healthy bodies and brains, and the nutrients we need to live longer and to live well. It's also devoid of the properties, phytochemicals, and longevity nutrients that have a broad range of functions in keeping us healthy.

This brings us to the paradox of the Healthy High-Tech Body. In order to enjoy the great benefits of modern science—the newest drugs and supplements, the advances in prevention and treatment protocols, the latest theories in fitness and exercise—we must always remember our roots: we are organic bodies responsive to the natural order of the animal kingdom.

We are products of evolution. Contrary to popular opinion (and wishful thinking), we have not evolved to be able to tolerate huge volumes of sugar and carbohydrates. We have not evolved to be able to consume huge portions of food at every sitting, simply because they are available. Having a Healthy High-Tech Body does not mean we can mistreat it, keep damaging it, and expect science to find ways for us to keep bouncing back. Reaching the pinnacle of High-Tech health means maintaining a tremendously well-performing body, in its best condition, fueled by foods that are appropriate for the human organism.

Food is the central hub around which everything else (healthwise) revolves. Like a sun with its satellite planets, everything in this book orbits around this section on food and the premises of what I call the Paleotech Diet.

"Paleo": The Principles
Behind the Paleotech Diet

The Paleotech Diet begins with the premise that our bodies and minds are adapted to the world and environment of hunter/gatherers that ended more than ten thousand years ago, with the advent of agriculture. According to Boyd Eaton, M.D., anthropologist and radiologist at Emory University in Atlanta, and the foremost authority on prehistoric (Paleolithic) diets, the human genome has changed little in the past forty thousand years. In fact, 99.9 percent of our genes date much farther back than forty thousand years and were therefore formed way before the development of agriculture. The implication is that our current ways of eating are "unfamiliar" to our genes and are causing malfunctions at every level of our health. The disparity between what we have been adapted to eat and what we are currently eating is making us older, fatter, and sicker than we should be.

Agriculture brought the cultivation of plant crops and cereal grains. Although cereal grains are the foundation of modern dietary guidelines worldwide, they have been central to the human diet for only "a moment" in our evolution. When we unite modern technologies of processing food with the marvels of present-day marketing, we are creating vast demands for foods that are packed with sugar and damaging fats, laced with hormone-disrupting chemicals, and bloated with calories. *Whew!*

Nobody expects you to eat only what cavemen ate. As Dr. Loren Cordain, an expert in Paleolithic nutrition at Colorado State University, says in an article called "The Paleolithic Diet and Its Modern Implications" (Designs for Health Institute, www.dfhl.com), "Clearly, humans can adapt to many types of diets. . . . However, our genetic constitution, including our nutritional requirement, was established in the remote past over eons of evolutionary experience. Human health and well-being can be optimized when we use the evolutionary paradigm as the starting point for present day nutrition."

Were we to eat in a way closer to what our bodies adapted to through eons of evolution, we'd all be better protected from the "diseases of affluence," including heart disease, adult-onset diabetes, and many types of cancer. *By merging the eating patterns of our ancestors with the best of modern science, we can design, advance, and engineer better, richer lives in a world that is vastly different from the one we were designed to inhabit.*

What we have done instead is create *antifoods* and *antinutrients* to fill our mouths and appetites, blowing our bodies up with them. The availability of these foods and their nufood compositions are launching people into lives of metabolic chaos.

Technology has provided the developed world with an unparalleled degree of comfort and convenience. We have created a consumer-oriented world of extraordinary novelty, filled with nufoods that have no nutritional purpose or value. We love to eat—which is important for our survival—but apparently we will eat just about anything, regardless of whether or not it is good for us.

WHAT WAS THAT WAY OF EATING? Before the advent of agriculture, all food was obtained by hunting and gathering. Our ancestors gathered fruits, roots, tubers, nuts, seeds, herbs, and vegetables. Everything you could hunt was fair game for eating—every kind of animal, including big and small game, fish, fowl, and eggs. Every morsel was eaten, including organs and brains. Insects and worms, good sources of protein, were also part of the diet. This diet was rich in what are called omega-3 essential fatty acids, which are critical to human health and are terribly deficient in today's diet. The diet provided a high volume of naturally occurring antioxidants, nutrients that protect us from many disease-causing agents.

With our modern palates and sensibilities, we're certainly not going to eat insects and worms. What we need is a rich and varied diet, high in "native foods," wonderfully prepared. Believe it or not, the Paleotech Diet embraces gourmet eating. In the next chapter, you'll find great ways of preparing healthy, species-appropriate food for breakfast, lunch, dinner, and snacks.

Willpower simply doesn't stand a chance when our ancestral instincts are telling us that we'd better eat as much as we can before the famine sets in—and when this new convenience-food environment makes it so easy for us to do so.

"Tech": Understanding the Food/Hormone Connection

Our ancestors did not have the kinds of food choices we have today. They didn't have breads, pastas, grain, and sugar-laden desserts. If they craved sweets, it was because they needed the vitamin C that fruits and berries provided. Whatever they consumed worked efficiently with their bodies' own chemistry.

The problem with today's modern diet is that much of it—the huge amounts of sugar and processed carbohydrates—does not react well with our bodies' chemistry, and, in fact, wreaks havoc with our health and well-being. That's because these nufood substances adversely affect chemicals, known as hormones, that are our bodies' biological messengers. They tell our organs, cells, and tissues what to do and when to do it. The hormonal (or endocrine) system is one of the body's great communications networks. Hormones are involved in just about every biological process: immune function, reproduction, growth, even controlling other hormones. And they work in extremely small concentrations—which is why it is so easy for even minute doses of harmful substances to disrupt their functioning efficiency and cause miscommunication.

This miscommunication within our highly complex bodies is what, according to Dr. Barry Sears, author of *The Zone*, causes much of modern illness and aging.

"Let's use the Internet as a metaphor for the body," says Dr. Sears. "We think of the Internet as a great testament to our technological brilliance—there are over 60 million people communicating information back and forth almost instantaneously, every day. Now let's look at our bodies. There are 60 *trillion* cells trying to communicate information back and forth almost instantaneously, every day. *This dwarfs the Internet!* Maybe we can look at modern illness and aging not as intrinsic diseases, but basically as just a case of information breakdown. If we can improve the information efficiency of our body we should be able to live longer and better lives."

What Does Insulin Do?

Insulin is one of two key hormones that, with its partner glucagon, direct the body's utilization of food for fuel. Insulin drives nutrients, primarily carbohydrates, into cells for immediate use or for future storage. Insulin is a storage hormone designed to take excess glucose (sugar) from dietary carbohydrates, excess amino acids from protein, and other nutrients, and store them as fat. It is a locking hormone; not only does it store fat, it locks it up so it can't be released.

Glucagon, insulin's biological opposite, is a mobilization hormone. It mobilizes stored energy (primarily carbohydrates) to be circulated in the bloodstream as a source of energy. Its primary job is to release stored carbohydrate, in the form of glucose, from the liver so that it can be used for energy.

An imbalance between these two hormones, usually seen as elevated insulin levels, can lead to the accumulation of body fat, promote diabetes, and speed up the development of heart disease.

What Does Cortisol Do?

Cortisol is a hormone produced in the adrenal glands that is critical to your body's ability to mediate stress. You have to be able to respond to any stressor, be it physical, biological, environmental, or even social, from overexertion to a viral infection to a screaming boss. Cortisol allows you to respond to different stressors in different ways. However, long-term exposure to unremitting stress (a boss who never stops screaming, a chaotic lifestyle that never slows down) will have dire consequences for your health, as too much cortisol can produce extensive biological damage and is a leading cause of premature aging. In addition, high levels of cortisol are a main factor in the loss of muscle and the accumulation of fat, especially around the stomach and gut area.

"Excess cortisol can be a nightmare," says Dr. Sears. "One of the greatest fears we have of aging is not disease—it's that our brain will give out before our body does. *And nothing will kill brain cells faster than excess cortisol.*"

Cortisol is perhaps the brain's greatest enemy. Your brain cells (neurons) are very sensitive to their environment; controlling this environment is your primary tool to prevent premature brain aging.

The brain requires glucose in order to survive. If inadequate glucose is getting to the brain, say as a function of poor regulation by the insulin/glucagon axis (which can happen easily if you're on a high-carbohydrate diet), then the brain will use cortisol as a backup system to get the fuel (glucose) it needs. There are vast numbers of brain cells that are easily damaged—if not outright killed—in the presence of excess cortisol. These cells are part of the brain called the hippocampus. When they die, so does your short-term memory.

Then, one imbalance leads to another. High carbohydrate consumption leads to high cortisol levels; high cortisol levels lead to brain malfunctions; brain malfunctions lead to increased stress, which leads to even higher levels of cortisol, and further acceleration of neuron loss and death. And so on and so on.

Scary, huh?

And Then There Are . . . Eicosanoids

There is a third group of hormones, called *eicosanoids*, that are secondary messengers in our bodies. They operate much like a traffic light signal system, dictating the flow of hormonal information by turning on a molecular green light for traffic to proceed in our bloodstream, or a molecular red light to stop the information flow. Eicosanoids are master hormones that control a wide range of physiological systems. When the signal system goes out of whack, so do many physiological systems. One group of "bad" eicosanoids can, for example, increase blood pressure. The primary cause of high "bad" eicosanoids is elevated insulin. If insulin is kept within its proper range, it will affect the production of "good" eicosanoids that keep our blood pressure normal. Eicosanoids have a hand in everything from inflammation and pain to how well your immune system works.

Hormonal Control: The First Step in the Paleotech Diet

So what can we do to maintain appropriate hormone levels? "There are three things you can do to control your hormones, and nobody else can do them for you," says Dr. Sears. "One is to watch what you eat. Two is to get enough exercise, and three is to reduce stress—to be sure you stop long enough to 'smell the roses' along the way."

Exercise and stress reduction will be covered under other pillars in this book, so for now we'll concentrate on the first, and most important, element in controlling your hormones—food.

In the context of the Healthy High-Tech Body, we want to help regulate the hardware—your body—and how well it can perform, by using the appropriate "software"—your food—to control:

- your insulin levels

- your cortisol levels

- your eicosanoid levels

The result will be the potential to control everything from the restoring and managing of your strength, your muscle mass, your stamina, and your sexuality, to decreasing your risk of degenerative illnesses.

THE GOLDEN RULES OF THE PALEOTECH DIET

1   Start with the "Paleo" dietary principles of our ancestors: fruits and vegetables rich in fiber and antioxidants; lean game, fish, and fowl; foods high in omega-3 fatty acids. (Of course, not all of our ancestors ate the same thing, just as not all cultures today eat the same foods. In places where few plants were available, our ancestors ate mostly animal protein. In places where edible plants were more abundant, prehistoric man ate the bulk of his food as carbohydrates. The human body is extremely adaptable in terms of what we are able to eat. However, the processed, additive-laden foods we eat today are quite different from the food that was available all those years ago.)

2   Incorporate the "tech" dietary principles based on our bodies' chemistry and hormonal systems: limit the amount of sugar, carbohydrates, and caffeine you consume. (These foods, in the forms that we find them today, were not available to the earliest societies of humans.)

3   Put these two sets of principles together and you've got the Golden Rules of the Paleotech Diet.

The Paleotech Diet

The U.S. government's official food pyramid tells you to base your diet on grains and carbohydrates. The Paleotech Diet asks you to take a lesson from your ancestors, turn that notion around, and base your diet on fiber-rich fruits and vegetables and lean proteins, with moderate servings of whole grains.

Your Paleotech Diet should adhere to the following practices:

Consume a high volume of fiber-rich/dense foods (at least six servings a day) Eat green leafy vegetables, such as spinach, watercress, lettuces (including mesclun), and a wide variety of sprouts. Add in vegetables like asparagus, peapods, tomatoes, carrots, zucchini, peppers, radishes, and cucumbers; cooked cruciferous vegetables, such as broccoli, kale, cauliflower, cabbage, and Brussels sprouts. Fiber also comes from seeds, nuts, and fruits—foods that figured prominently in the Paleolithic diet. Note that your risk of stroke drops *6 percent* for every serving of veggies and fruits you have a day (topping off at six servings). We're talking about a higher than 30 percent reduction, compared with diets containing three or fewer servings. And, according to the American Heart Institute and research from the Framingham Heart Study, the ongoing Nurses Health Study, and the Professionals Follow-up Study, there are well over 1.1 million heart attacks in America each year, with a 40 percent fatality rate. On the other hand, high fiber intake is associated with a 40 to 50 percent *reduction* in the risk of cardiovascular disease and heart attack.

Many studies show that higher intakes of fruits and vegetables are also associated with lower risks of cancer. Prostate cancer risks appear to be lower for men who consume twenty-eight or more servings of veggies per week. And, as part of a study of 124,000 men and women, researchers found that people with the greatest intake of a group of nutrients called "mixed carotenoids," indicating a diverse vegetable and fruit intake, were 32 percent less likely to develop lung cancer, as compared with those who consumed few carotenoids. Nonsmokers with a high consumption of "alpha-carotene" (a relative of beta-carotene) had a 63 percent lower risk of lung cancer, and lycopene, a nutrient found in tomatoes, was associated with a 27 percent reduced risk of lung cancer among smokers.

A TEA BREAK **Green Tea,** which originated in China four hundred years ago, can help protect against cancer and heart disease. It may also strengthen bones in postmenopausal women.

In a study of more than 35,000 women published in the *American Journal of Epidemiology* (1996; 44:175–182), women who drank two cups of green tea were 68 percent less likely to develop cancer of the digestive tract and 40 percent less likely to develop urinary tract cancer.

According to a British study published in the *American Journal of Clinical Nutrition* (2000; 71:1003–1007), women aged sixty-five to seventy-five who drank one cup of tea daily had higher bone density in both their spines and their thighs.

Other studies show that tea may turn out to be a potent weapon against cancers of the stomach, prostate, esophagus, and bladder.

Drink up!

Consume fruits that are rich in natural antioxidants and vitamin C Blueberries and strawberries, for instance, are rich in antioxidants. Blueberries have been shown to improve both coordination and short-term memory, according to a United States Department of Agriculture study. Besides being potent antioxidants, they have anti-inflammatory and blood-thinning effects. I can't recommend them enough.

Apples are rich in naturally occurring antioxidants known as phenolics and flavonoids. Apparently these antioxidants, along with other nutrients found in apples (especially unpeeled apples), provide protection against cancer, as demonstrated in a Cornell University study showing the inhibition of colon and liver cancer cells using these nutrients.

Research shows that a compound called resviratol, found in some nuts, berries, grapes (especially red grapes), raspberries, and peanuts (if you're not allergic to them), fights both cancer and heart disease and reduces inflammation.

Consume foods rich in omega-3 fatty acids Here's some healthy advice: eat fish, fish, and more fish—salmon, sardines, halibut, tuna, mackerel, bass, swordfish, mahi-mahi, cod, trout, and shellfish, such as crab and shrimp.

Olive oil, fish oil, certain nuts, and seeds (and their respective oils) also provide this extraordinary nutrient.

In an attempt to reduce the amount of fat in their diets, including saturated fats and cholesterol, Americans have also succeeded in reducing all the great sources of omega-3 fatty acids. This rush to eliminate fats, along with an increase in consumed carbohydrates, has been a central source of many health imbalances affecting our brain's performance. Looking at our evolution, we see evidence that the high consumption of omega-3 food sources, especially fish, may have played a role in the growth, development, and evolution of the cerebral cortex. The consumption of fish-based omega-3 fats may have boosted our ancestors' intelligence as well.

More recent evidence shows that a deficiency of DHA (a component of omega-3 fats) during pregnancy can impair a modern child's intelligence and visual acuity, as well as being a contributing factor to depression and possibly even attention deficit disorder. A five-year study at the National Institute of Alcoholism and Alcohol Abuse, the University of Antwerp in Belgium, the University of Sheffield, England, and other institutions found that depressed people have exaggerated immune responses coupled with deficient levels of omega-3 fatty acids. This has led investigators to believe that low levels of omega-3 fatty acids may actually play a key role in depression. In a cross-national analysis, the prevalence of major depression is sixty times lower in countries where fish is consumed daily! Further, a comprehensive study of two hundred elderly subjects showed that low blood levels of DHA were a predictor of greater symptoms of depression and anxiety, and in a nine-year study of a thousand people, those with high DHA levels were more than 40 percent less likely to develop dementia (including Alzheimer's disease) than people with low

GO NUTS The best nuts for snacking and to use as condiments (because of their high-quality fats and oils) are walnuts, pecans, macadamias, pine nuts, hazelnuts, and almonds. These are rich sources of omega-3 fatty acids. Even better, roast them a bit to make their nutrients more bioavailable.

THE CHOLESTEROL CONUNDRUM We have been taught over the past few decades that red meat, fats, and especially eggs contain cholesterol and therefore should be avoided. But the latest data tell us that we may have been too quick to judge.

Cholesterol is actually essential to our survival. It helps produce vitamin D and helps the body repair damaged cell membranes. It is a building block for estrogen and testosterone, and is necessary for the production of cortisone. Cholesterol is divided into "good" and "bad" cholesterol. "Good," or HDL, cholesterol is carried to the liver, broken down into bile, and eventually eliminated from the body. "Bad," or LDL, cholesterol carries fat and cholesterol throughout the body and deposits them in various spots, including the arteries (which impedes or prevents blood flow to the heart).

If you greatly reduce the amount of cholesterol you're ingesting, the body will only produce more. So the warnings we've been given about eating cholesterol don't seem to hold up. And once again, insulin enters into the equation. When you eat a high-carbohydrate, high-sugar diet, you increase the level of insulin in the body, which signals the cells to produce more cholesterol. The excess cholesterol that is then produced builds up in the arteries. If you follow the guidelines of the Paleotech Diet, you will automatically reduce the level of insulin, and therefore the level of excess cholesterol, in your body.

levels of DHA. Therefore, it seems likely that an increase in severity of depression indicates a lower consumption of omega-3 fats.

Omega-3 fatty acids are also the building blocks of the body's anti-inflammatory eicosanoids, the ones that control inflammatory damage to tissue. A study done on the traditional Greek diet found that the high consumption of olive oil reduced the risk of rheumatoid arthritis (inflammation of the joints). The study, appearing in the *Journal of Clinical Nutrition* (1999; 70:1077–1082), associated both the consumption of olive oil and cooked vegetables with a 61 percent reduced risk of having the disease.

Choose lean protein As stated earlier, many of our prehistoric ancestors ate high-protein diets. However, it would be almost impossible for modern humans to re-create such a diet. The animal protein they consumed was quite different from the animal protein found in today's supermarkets. The meat our ancestors consumed came from animals that grazed and hunted in the wild. It was exceptionally lean and muscular (think about it: those animals spent their lives running from predators). The meat was also high in unsaturated fats, such as omega-3 fatty acid. There was very little saturated fat (the kind that leads to clogged arteries and heart disease). The meat we eat today, mostly beef, comes from grain-fed animals. It is full of saturated fat.

You can certainly find lean meat today if you shop carefully. You can buy meat from animals that are range fed, meaning that they graze on available grasses. Although red meat has gotten a bad rap in years past, beef contains two and one half times the iron of chicken. Iron is an essential mineral, especially for women, and so is zinc, which is found in both pork and beef. Chicken, turkey, eggs, and mozzarella, feta, cottage, and farmer cheeses are also good sources of protein.

Choose whole grains and minimize the consumption of cereal grains or grain products Melvin Konner, co-author of *The Paleolithic Prescription,* stated in an article in the *Washington Post* called "Stone Age Soup" (February 13, 2001) that there is no reason grains shouldn't be a substantial part of our diet. The problem, however, is that "what we do with grains is refine them until there's no fiber, no vitamin and mineral content." The grains that we do eat in pasta, cereals, bread, and bagels are frequently high in *gluten*, which is found primarily in wheat and wheat-based products. Gluten, which is a portion of the grain that is difficult for many people to assimilate, has been linked to a large number of physical disorders, from arthritis to schizophrenia. A plethora of digestive disorders, from bloating and gas to celiac disease, are also linked to an inability to handle this nutrient. There may be a whole host of immune disorders, including depression, high blood pressure, eczema, and psoriasis, that are associated with the consumption of gluten-rich foods.

This is not an isolated problem. Many people who suffer from gluten intolerance to some degree don't even know it. It's only when they stop eating it that they notice how much better they feel.

Eat only grains, beans, and root vegetable carbohydrates that register low on the glycemic index The *glycemic index* is designed to measure how rapidly a carbohydrate is absorbed into your bloodstream and its potential impact on insulin secretion. The higher a food's glycemic value, the faster it enters the bloodstream. When that happens, the pancreas responds by secreting insulin. While that does bring blood sugar levels down, it also "tells" the body to store fat and keep it stored up. Over time this will not only make you fat, it will keep you fat.

Note that the absorption of carbohydrates can be slowed down if you ingest fat (for example, fish oil, olive oil, sesame oil, or butter) along with them. For instance, if you eat fish (which, obviously, contains fish oil) with rice on the side, the oil modifies the glycemic "impact" of the rice on your bloodstream, or the rate of its conversion and absorption into blood sugar.

Foods on the glycemic index are scored on a scale of 0 to 100, 100 being the absolute value of pure glucose (sugar). The lower the glycemic value of a food, the better. The higher the value, the closer it gets to pure sugar in your blood (very bad).

Here is a list of sixteen carbohydrates and their glycemic values. If you're eating carbs, try and choose from this list—just remember that if you choose a food with a high value (such as couscous), you should eat it with a moderate amount of fat in order to reduce its glycemic impact.

Contents from the *Glucose Revolution* Top 100 Low Glycemic Foods

Food	Glycemic Score
1. black beans	30
2. chickpeas	33
3. chana dal bean	8
4. red kidney beans	27
5. lentils	30
6. basmati rice	58
7. brown rice	55
8. sweet potato	54
9. taro	54
10. yam	51
11. oats	49
12. barley	25
13. kasha	54
14. couscous	65
15. peas (split, dried, yellow, green)	22
16. maize (corn)	55

The above choices are from three categories of starchy foods: the bean-legume family, grains, and starchy root vegetables. It is not an exhaustive list, nor definitive. It is, rather, a group of carbohydrates that I find acceptable as part of the Paleotech Diet.

The Paleotech Diet is rich in a wide variety of plant foods and vegetables; fruits, seeds, and nuts; a modest amount of lean, high-quality meats, such as poultry (including eggs) and occasional lean cuts of red meat; lots of omega-3 fatty acid–rich seafood; oils from a variety of plant sources; and a modest amount of grains and root vegetables.

Paleotech Diet Enhancers

As you read on through the chapters of this book, you'll come across one word over and over again: efficiency. A Healthy High-Tech Body is built by increasing the efficiency of all its systems. The Paleotech Diet increases the efficiency of your hormonal system. If you want to further enhance that efficiency, you can add two more High-Tech elements to your diet: longevity nutrients and organic foods.

Longevity nutrients As the technology of food has progressed over the twentieth and into the twenty-first century, there has been more and more research into its nourishing properties. One of the newest categories is *longevity nutrients,* found in a wide variety of foods. These longevity nutrients protect against the development of diabetes, decrease blood sugar, regulate insulin, and reduce the risk of cardiovascular heart disease and stroke. Some of these nutrients, with strange-sounding names such as glucosinolates, indoles, phenols, dithilthiones, protease inhibitors, allium compounds, and limonene, have complementary and overlapping relationships that include everything from binding carcinogenic agents in the digestive system (aiding your body in the detoxification and removal of destructive chemicals), to regulating hormones, to offering antioxidant and anti-aging effects.

In his book *The New Longevity Diet,* Dr. Henry Mallek has done a great job of codifying these nutrients, identifying where in the diet they show up and of what benefit they are to us. They appear to be more complex and have greater ranges of function than many vitamins and minerals. Here are a few of them:

Nucleotides: found in animal protein sources, especially fish. Nucleotides are the building blocks of DNA (DNA is made up of nucleic acids, which are composed of nucleotides). Research indicates that we need 450 to 700 milligrams of nucleotides daily to provide continued support to the immune system, which declines as we age. Nucleotides help to repair the lining of our digestive and intestinal tracts, the cells of which are rebuilt and replaced every three to six days.

Saponins: found in legumes and beans, they are critical for enhanced immune performance. They work to lower cholesterol and prevent cancer.

Protease inhibitors: found in foods ranging from spinach to peaches, corn, and sweet potatoes, these nutrients appear to protect DNA from malfunctioning. They may also protect against various cancers, such as colon, breast, and prostate cancer. In addition, they appear to have anti-aging effects.

Carnosine: a member of the exorphin family, found only in animal protein—lamb, poultry, wild game—carnosine protects the brain from free-radical damage. It also slows down wrinkling and keeps connective tissue from aging. This is a *top gun antioxidant.* Other exorphins called cyclic peptides, found in tuna and shrimp, help regulate digestion and are used by the brain for appetite control.

Monoterpines: master detoxifiers found in citrus fruits, they selectively seek out harmful substances in the blood that can lead to malignant cell overgrowth. They can also slow down malignant tumors that have already developed. Monoterpines prevent carcinogens and other toxic chemicals from interacting with DNA. They interact with proteins that signal cell death, making them invaluable in the prevention of aging.

Eating according to the Paleotech Diet will provide many of these nutrients naturally.

The organic connection   *Important High-Tech longevity note*: try to eat "organically" whenever you can. Organic foods are free of synthetic pesticides and chemicals, artificial additives, and preservatives. Animals and poultry must be fed only organic feed: no growth hormones and no systematically applied antibiotics.

Eating organically can help ensure that the foods you consume still contain active longevity nutrients. It can also reduce the buildup of chemicals in your body, which can adversely affect your hormonal communications. Many of the chemicals that are added to our foods are called *hormone disruptors*. They can interfere with the development and functioning of our body systems. A hormone disruptor acts like a wrench tossed into your metabolic engine. Many disruptors actually mimic hormones, turning gene signals on and off and creating disturbances that can throw your metabolic balance off at any given point. Additives run the gamut from growth-promoting hormones and antibiotics (twenty-five million pounds a year at last count) to pesticides, herbicides, and substances that modify food (such as coloring agents, texturizers, and flavor enhancers). I'll discuss how to "cleanse" your body of these toxins in the upcoming chapter on detoxification.

The good news is that eating organically even part-time can provide surprising benefits. For instance, in her book *Hormone Deception,* Lindsey Berkson cites a study of male Danish organic farmers, showing that those who ate organic food just 25 percent of the time had a 43 percent higher sperm count.

Paleotech Diet Don'ts

Beware the overconsumption of sugar and carbohydrates After years of eating breads, pastas, noodles, cakes, cookies, pizzas, muffins, cereal, and refined sugars, the tissues in our bodies become rigid and pigmented (producing age spots) with deposits of tissue-stiffening compounds called Advanced Glycation End Products, or AGEs. The overconsumption of sugar and carbohydrates, in all their forms, produce these "stiff sugar protein bonds," which accumulate in our bodies as we get older. These bonds are a result of sugar "gluing" itself to our collagen, veins, arteries, ligaments, bones, *brains*, you name it, producing a constellation of changes, including stiff joints, hardened arteries, failing organs, and enfeebled muscles. Sugar will combine with almost anything. It's extremely sticky—just think of sugar drying on your fingers. Sugar-driven damage accumulates as we age and accelerates the deterioration of *all* our functions and capabilities. Not only is increased glycation unhealthy, it speeds up the wrinkling of your skin and makes you look older than you are.

Here are some facts about sugar:

- Sugar consumption in 1821 was ten pounds per person per year. Currently, it's about 150 pounds per person per year (noncaloric sweeteners add another 50 pounds per person per year).

- Pepsi-Cola contains 1.2 teaspoons of sugar per ounce of soda. Most cans contain twelve ounces.

- Pepsi-Cola spent $200 million in advertising in the year 2000. Coke spent $300 million.

- Quaker Instant Oatmeal, cinnamon or spice-flavored, packs 4.3 teaspoons of sugar per ounce.

- Heinz Custard Pudding (baby food) contains four teaspoons of sugar. Why?

- Ounce-per-ounce, most breakfast cereals contain more sugar than a soft drink. Count among them Honeycomb cereal, Froot Loops, Cocoa Puffs, etc.

Longevity nutrients are part of the Paleotech Diet and are essential to maintaining health. As you can see from this chapter, food is a central force in shaping the architecture of your health, vitality, immunity, weight, appearance, emotionality, and possibly the length of your life. The Paleotech Diet is the foundation on which you can build a great supplement program to enrich and deepen your results. The Paleotech Diet is the foundation for reaping the maximum benefits of an exercise program. If you want the maximum results from the other sections in this book, begin making these dietary changes. Incorporate them at a speed you can handle, but the quicker the better. Marrying this section to selected products in the Power Brain chapter, for example, will give you exponentially better results if you want to prevent brain aging, increase intelligence, and improve memory.

In her book *The Crazy Makers*, Carol Simontacchi writes, "When large amounts of sugar flood the bloodstream, the body reacts by releasing insulin from the pancreas to keep blood sugar levels within a narrow range. Both excessive and large amounts of sugar damage the brain. When huge amounts of sugar are consumed over the course of a lifetime, the pancreas loses its ability to regulate blood sugar levels precisely, often overreacting to the presence of sugar . . . this condition is called 'carbohydrate sensitivity.' . . . Growing evidence suggests that carbohydrate sensitivity is a common problem leading to a number of health disorders, including diabetes and heart disease."

Limit caffeine intake For many people coffee appears to just fry their brains. In small amounts, once in a while, I see no problem; in fact, there appears to be some connection between moderate caffeine use and a protective effect on the brain against Alzheimer's and Parkinson's diseases. However, many people don't know the meaning of "moderate" caffeine use and are altering everything from their moods to their sleeping patterns with the high consumption of caffeine.

Too much coffee can contribute to depression, anxiety, and insomnia. It seems that as it raises the energy metabolism throughout the brain by increasing the stimulating neurohormones noradrenaline and dopamine, it also *reduces* the amount of blood flowing to the brain. At the same time, it reduces the levels of the calming neurotransmitter serotonin. This is one hell of a bind. (Think of all the people using powerful drugs such as Prozac or Zoloft, which are designed to increase levels of serotonin in the brain, washing their meds down in the morning with a cup of coffee. What does that do, when these two conflicting forces are pulpifying your brain, as you begin your workday?)

Coffee also raises blood pressure, increasing the risk of heart disease. In a study of twelve thousand men and women in Norway, the higher the consumption of coffee, the higher the levels found in the blood of a deadly amino acid known as homocysteine. Homocysteine promotes hardening of the arteries, increasing the risk of a heart attack. Coffee increases the amounts and effects of cortisol in the body (and we already know what long-term exposure to excessive cortisol will do to us).

Now you know the principles behind the Paleotech Diet. If you follow none of the other advice throughout this book, you'll still be well on your way to High-Tech health. If you're thinking that the Paleotech Diet is dull or restrictive in any way, turn to the next chapter for some delicious, healthy recipes your ancestors never enjoyed.

3 The Paleotech Gourmet

Recipes for High-Tech nutritional health

In their search for fitness and longevity, many health-conscious people are willing to make major changes in their lives because they believe that science has all the answers. They go to the gym and use the latest ergonomically designed equipment. They take multivitamins and herbal supplements. They keep up on the most recent breakthroughs in medical and pharmaceutical treatments.

It seems, however, that when it comes to food most people have the greatest difficulty changing their habits and lifestyles. It's difficult to think of food as a High-Tech solution to anything, it's such a low-tech part of our daily maintenance. However, if you follow the Paleotech Diet guidelines, you're automatically applying High-Tech, scientific solutions to many of your health-related problems.

The recipes and meal suggestions that follow in this chapter adhere closely to those guidelines. For the most part, they do not include much sugar or starchy carbohydrates. Every day, Americans are bombarded with carbohydrates; it often seems that carbs make up "all the good stuff." However, health problems are created when we eat too many of the wrong kind of carbohydrates, not only because they're innately unhealthy but also because when we're eating these huge amounts of carbs, we're not eating enough fats and proteins. And when we don't get enough fat and protein, we create major problems in controlling our hormones, as discussed in chapter 2.

On the other hand, foods that follow the Paleotech guidelines help regulate insulin and cortisol, reduce inflammation in the body, and provide appropriate amounts of fiber and omega-3 fatty acids.

The Paleotech Gourmet recipes have been created by Dr. Deborah Chud (a physician as well as a gourmet cook), author of *The Gourmet Prescription*. All of the recipes included here are based on her knowledge of how foods affect our health and well-being.

"Protein, fat, and fiber act as brakes on the insulin production machine," says Dr. Chud, "because they slow down the digestion of food. The slower our food is digested, the more gradually our blood sugar rises, and the slower the production of insulin. This lowers the average insulin level throughout the day, which is the ultimate goal."

However, it doesn't matter how healthy a meal may be if it doesn't appeal to our senses. Most "diets" present meals that are restricting, constricting, and just plain boring. But to Dr. Chud, food has to be "exciting." She keeps that in mind whenever she cooks.

"Think about it. Starchy foods—potatoes and rice and pizza dough—the high-glycemic carbs, are not the flavor-bearing elements of food. Pasta all by itself doesn't have much flavor, nor do potatoes or rice. It's the sauces and the seasonings that give these foods their taste. Once I realized that, I knew I could still have highly flavored foods without suffering the consequences of eating a high-carbohydrate, high-glycemic meal. I could just eliminate the offending substances and develop recipes that retain all of the flavor and sophistication of the foods I used to eat."

These are dishes that will keep you healthy and satisfied throughout the day.

All-Purpose Flavor Enhancers

Slow-Roasted Plum Tomatoes

These roasted tomatoes contain twice as much carbohydrate per cup as fresh tomatoes, but much more than twice the flavor. Use them as a side dish with grilled chicken, lamb, beef, or fish, or as a component in sautés, stews, omelets, and frittatas. Feel free to substitute them for fresh tomatoes, but remember to halve the quantity to keep the carbohydrate counts the same.

MAKES 2 CUPS

> 2½ pounds plum tomatoes, cored and halved lengthwise
> Kosher salt
> Chopped fresh herbs (optional)

1   Preheat the oven to 200 degrees. Spray a nonstick baking sheet with olive oil. Place the tomatoes on the baking sheet, cut side up, and season generously with salt. Sprinkle with fresh herbs, if desired. Roast for 4 to 6 hours until the edges of the tomatoes have shriveled but they remain juicy. They should lose about 50 percent of their weight by the end of roasting, but should not become hard, dry, or blackened.

2   Use immediately or store the tomatoes in an airtight container in the refrigerator for 5 to 6 days.

TOMATO FACTS Many recent studies have discovered that tomatoes are a potent antioxidant. They are a great source of lycopene, an antioxidant substance that gives tomatoes their luscious red color. Tomatoes supply up to 90 percent of the lycopene most of us get in our diet. In order to receive the most benefit, tomatoes should be cooked and combined with fats such as olive oil.

Roasted Garlic Paste

Roasted garlic paste has manifold uses in sauces, salad dressings, and marinades. Its full, mellow flavor gives depth to many dishes without the sharp bite and lingering aftertaste of raw garlic. Natural antibacterial properties make it highly resistant to spoilage. Freeze it in small, airtight containers and defrost only what you need.

MAKES 1 CUP

> 4 large garlic bulbs, preferably with large cloves
> 1 teaspoon extra virgin olive oil
> 4 to 6 tablespoons water

1 Remove the loose papery outer skin from the garlic bulbs without dislodging the cloves. Cut off the top ¼ inch of each bulb. Place 1 garlic bulb, cut side up, in the center of a 10-inch square of aluminum foil. Drizzle with ¼ teaspoon oil. Fold the foil to make a closed packet. Set in a baking dish. Repeat with the remaining bulbs. (Alternatively, you may roast the garlic in a terra-cotta roaster following the manufacturer's instructions.)

2 Turn the oven to 300 degrees (do not preheat). Roast for 30 minutes. Remove the garlic from the foil and return to the baking dish. Roast for 45 minutes.

3 When the bulbs are cool enough to handle, separate the cloves and squeeze them out of their skins. Place the peeled cloves in a food processor. With the motor running, add 4 tablespoons water. Process until smooth, scraping down the sides as needed. Add more water if necessary. The paste will keep for 3 weeks in an airtight container in the refrigerator or for up to 6 months in the freezer.

GARLIC FACTS Garlic is one of the oldest known medicinal herbs. It was worshiped by the ancient Egyptians and chewed by Greek Olympic athletes (and has long been known to keep vampires away). It's the sulfur-containing compounds that give garlic its pungent aroma as well as many of its healing properties. Garlic has been shown to lower cholesterol and blood pressure. It also stimulates the immune system and may be particularly effective in treating upper-respiratory viral infections. This amazing food also contains selenium, an antioxidant that protects cell membranes and DNA from damage and helps neutralize carcinogens and other toxins.

Basic Marinara Sauce

A first-rate marinara is a marvelous thing. It makes an Italian entrée out of shellfish with almost no effort and instantly transforms vegetables like eggplant into hearty, flavorful side dishes. For convenience, store it in airtight 2-cup containers. It will keep for at least a week in the refrigerator or for up to 6 months in the freezer.

MAKES 8 TO 10 CUPS

1 tablespoon plus 1 teaspoon extra virgin olive oil

3 tablespoons minced garlic

3 tablespoons minced flat-leaf parsley

¼ to ½ teaspoon hot red pepper flakes

Three 35-ounce cans Italian plum tomatoes with their liquid, basil leaf removed

1 to 1½ teaspoons kosher salt

Freshly ground black pepper

Heat the oil in a large, deep nonstick skillet over medium heat. Add the garlic, parsley, and red pepper flakes. Sauté for 2 minutes. Add the tomatoes and their juice. Bring to a simmer. Using a potato masher, gently crush the tomatoes without splattering the juice. Simmer for 1½ hours, uncovered, until thick. Add the salt and pepper to taste. Serve immediately.

Basic Roquefort Dressing

Pureed tofu can serve as a healthy, low-carbohydrate base for many rich-tasting dips and dressings. By combining it with other ingredients (e.g., nonfat yogurt or buttermilk, low-fat sour cream or mayonnaise), you can alter texture and flavor. Extra tofu yields a thicker consistency, ideal for dips. A little nonfat buttermilk creates a tangier, thinner blend, perfect for ranch dressing. Add mayonnaise and yogurt for cole slaw dressings. Add sour cream and yogurt for Green Goddess, cucumber-dill, and horseradish sauces. Conduct your own experiments. Try Basic Roquefort Dressing on salad greens and with crudités.

1 cup pureed low-fat silken tofu

¼ cup nonfat plain yogurt

¼ cup low-fat sour cream

3 tablespoons tarragon vinegar

2 teaspoons anchovy paste

2 teaspoons Roasted Garlic Paste
  (page 62)

3 ounces Roquefort cheese, crumbled

¼ cup minced flat-leaf parsley

½ teaspoon kosher salt

Freshly ground black pepper

Combine the tofu, yogurt, sour cream, vinegar, anchovy paste, and roasted garlic paste in a bowl or measuring cup. Whisk vigorously to blend. (You can also use a food processor.) Add the Roquefort, parsley, salt, and pepper to taste and stir to combine. Store in the refrigerator for up to 1 week.

TOFU FACTS Tofu, also known as soybean curd, was first used in China around 200 B.C. In recipes it acts like a sponge and soaks up whatever flavors surround it. There are three basic kinds of tofu: firm, soft, and silken. Firm is fairly solid and is good in stir-fries, soups, and on the grill. This type of tofu is highest in protein, fat, and calcium content. Soft tofu is good in Oriental soups and in recipes that call for blending. Silken tofu is creamy and custardlike and works well in pureed or blended dishes like this one. Soy is a great source of protein and essential fatty acids. It has been shown to inhibit both breast and prostate cancer, lower cholesterol, and help prevent osteoporosis.

Basic Balsamic Vinaigrette

This dressing keeps indefinitely in the refrigerator. If the oil solidifies, liquefy it by gently warming it in the microwave. Shake well immediately before each use.

  6 tablespoons best-quality commercial balsamic vinegar

  6 tablespoons water

  2 tablespoons Dijon mustard

  2 tablespoons extra virgin olive oil

Combine the vinegar, water, mustard, and oil in a salad cruet or jar. Shake well. Refrigerate until ready to serve. Bring to room temperature and shake well before use.

Roasted Fennel with Herbes de Provence and Garlic

Herbes de Provence contains both French and Italian herbs: savory, rosemary, cracked fennel, thyme, basil, tarragon, lavender, and marjoram. Vegetable dishes as well as roasted meats and poultry benefit from its aromatic influence. It is available from Penzeys Spices (800-741-8878 or www.penzeys.com).

MAKES 4 SERVINGS

  4 large fennel bulbs, stalks removed, fronds reserved

  1 tablespoon extra virgin olive oil

  2 teaspoons minced garlic

  1 teaspoon Herbes de Provence

  Salt and freshly ground black pepper

1 Preheat the oven to 450 degrees. Halve the fennel bulbs lengthwise and remove the cores. Place the cut sides of each bulb together and wrap each bulb tightly in an aluminum foil packet. Arrange the packets on a baking sheet and roast for 40 minutes until

tender. When cool enough to handle, remove from the packets, drain, and cut lengthwise into ⅓-inch slices. Do not be concerned if the layers of the slices separate. (The fennel can be prepared to this point up to 3 days in advance and refrigerated.)

2 Chop the fronds and reserve 2 tablespoons for garnish. Set aside the remainder for another use.

FENNEL FACTS Fennel, with its delicate licorice taste, is a great flavor enhancer. It has a broad, bulbous base, a celerylike stem and bright green feathery leaves. It can be eaten raw or cooked in a variety of ways. Fennel is an excellent source of vitamin A, and also contains a fair amount of calcium, phosphorus, and potassium.

3 Heat the oil in a large nonstick skillet over medium heat. Add the garlic and herbs and sauté for 1 minute. Add the fennel and season generously with salt and pepper. Toss with 2 wooden spatulas for several minutes until heated through. Serve immediately, garnished with fronds.

Breakfast Treats

Mixed Berry Bowl with Apricot Cream

Pureed silken tofu boosts the protein content of the cottage cheese in this refreshing breakfast treat. This recipe lends itself to endless variations: the apricot cream is delicious on many other fruits (peaches, plums, and cherries work well), and the cream itself may be varied with different fruit preserves (blackberry, red currant, strawberry, and blueberry are all excellent).

MAKES 4 SERVINGS

2 cups low-fat cottage cheese

2 cups pureed low-fat silken tofu, about 1 pound

4 tablespoons no-sugar-added apricot preserves
   or spoon fruit

2 cups sliced strawberries

2 cups raspberries

2 cups blueberries

3 tablespoons sliced or slivered almonds, toasted

1   Combine the cottage cheese and pureed tofu in a food processor and process until smooth. Transfer to a bowl. Add the preserves and whisk to blend. (The apricot cream may be prepared up to 3 days in advance and refrigerated.)

2   Divide the berries among 4 bowls and spoon the apricot cream over them. Sprinkle with the almonds and serve immediately.

BERRY FACTS Berries are among the healthiest foods you can eat. Not only do they have incredible antioxidant properties, they are packed full of insoluble fiber (especially in those tiny seeds that get stuck between your teeth), which helps protect against heart disease.

Huevos Rancheros
with Black Beans

From the perspective of insulin control, home-cooked beans are superior to canned because they have a lower glycemic index. In other words, they provoke a smaller insulin response. Coincidentally, they have far better flavor and texture. Although they are time-consuming to make, dried beans can be cooked in large batches and stored in small quantities in the freezer for up to 6 months. When they are cool, simply drain them and transfer 1 or 2 cups at a time to small Ziploc bags. Push out the air and seal. Defrost overnight in the refrigerator or in minutes in the microwave. Once you've tasted them, you'll never use canned beans again!

MAKES 3 SERVINGS

    1 tablespoon plus ½ teaspoon extra virgin olive oil

    1 cup chopped onion

    ½ cup chopped red bell pepper

    ½ cup chopped yellow bell pepper

    ½ cup chopped green bell pepper

    1 tablespoon minced garlic

    ½ teaspoon ground cumin

    ½ teaspoon chili powder

    ½ teaspoon oregano

    ¼ teaspoon hot red pepper flakes

    3 cups chopped fresh tomatoes, or one 28-ounce can diced tomatoes, briefly drained

    2 cups cooked or canned black beans, drained

    1 teaspoon salt plus more for the eggs

    Freshly ground black pepper

    Tabasco sauce

    3 whole eggs

    12 egg whites

1   Heat the oil in a large nonstick skillet over medium heat. Add the onion, peppers, garlic, cumin, chili powder, oregano, and red pepper flakes. Cook for 5 minutes, or until soft, stirring occasionally. Stir in the tomatoes, beans, 1 teaspoon salt, pepper, and Tabasco to taste. Bring to a boil and simmer, uncovered, for 10 minutes, or until nearly all of the liquid has evaporated.

2   Gently drop the whole eggs onto the simmering vegetable-bean mixture at some distance from each other. Fill in the intervening space with the egg whites. Season with salt and pepper. Cover and cook for 6 to 8 minutes, or until the whites are opaque and the yolks are cooked to desired doneness. Divide the eggs and vegetable-bean mixture among 3 plates and serve immediately.

BEAN FACTS History shows that humans have been eating beans for more than ten thousand years. The ancient Greeks held bean feasts to honor the god Apollo, and Egyptians put beans in the pharaohs' tombs for an afterlife snack. Beans add valuable fiber to your diet, but they also contain a high amount of what's called resistant starch, a substance that helps clean out your system and promote bowel health. Beans also contain anticancer compounds called phytates and protease inhibitors. They pack more protein than any other plant food, plus zinc, potassium, magnesium, calcium, and iron. They're also rich in folic acid, which helps depress homocysteine, an amino acid that promotes clogged arteries and heart disease. Beans also help stabilize blood sugar. Eating beans produces a slow rise in blood sugar, which means you produce less insulin. A rise in insulin triggers hunger; therefore, if you eat beans at breakfast or lunch, you're less likely to overeat later in the day.

Creamed Trout Toasts with Apple

Chickpea flour contains considerably less carbohydrate and more fiber per table-spoon than wheat flour. It also has a lower glycemic index. It is available in health food stores and from Bob's Red Mill Natural Foods, Inc. (503-654-3215 or www.bobsredmill.com).

MAKES 4 SERVINGS

> 1 pound smoked trout
>
> 2 teaspoons neutral oil, such as canola, or butter
>
> 2 tablespoons chickpea flour
>
> 1½ cups skim milk
>
> ½ cup pureed low-fat silken tofu
>
> 2 tablespoons minced flat-leaf parsley (optional)
>
> ¼ teaspoon kosher salt
>
> Freshly ground black pepper
>
> 6 slices whole grain rye or pumpernickel bread
>
> 3 Granny Smith apples, cored and thinly sliced

1 Remove the skin and bones from the trout and flake into a bowl. (You should have about 12 ounces of fish, or approximately 2 cups.)

2 Heat the oil or butter in a saucepan over medium heat. Add the chickpea flour and whisk continuously for 30 seconds. Remove from the heat and whisk in the milk. Return to medium heat and bring the milk to a boil. Boil gently for 5 minutes, whisking occasionally. Adjust the heat so that the milk does not boil over. Whisk in the tofu and remove from the heat. Stir in the trout, parsley (if using), salt, and black pepper to taste. (The sauce can be prepared up to 24 hours in advance and refrigerated. Warm in a saucepan or in the microwave before serving.)

3 Meanwhile, toast the bread until very crisp and cut in half. Arrange the slices on a broiler pan and divide the apple slices among them. Spoon the warm sauce over the apples. Broil 3 inches from the flame for 1 to 2 minutes until lightly browned. Serve immediately.

Pepper Frittata with Garlic Chives

Garlic chives are available in Asian markets. If you cannot find them, substitute regular chives and a little garlic.

Makes 3 servings

> 1 tablespoon extra virgin olive oil
>
> 1 cup garlic chives in 1-inch lengths,
>   or 1 cup regular chives and 1 teaspoon minced garlic
>
> 3 whole eggs
>
> 12 egg whites
>
> ¼ cup grated Parmesan cheese
>
> 1 teaspoon kosher salt
>
> Freshly ground black pepper
>
> ¾ cup julienned roasted red bell peppers
>
> ¾ cup julienned roasted yellow bell peppers
>
> Olive oil spray
>
> 3 large beefsteak tomatoes, thickly sliced
>
> 3 slices pumpernickel

1 Preheat the oven to 450 degrees. Heat 1 teaspoon of the oil in a large ovenproof nonstick skillet over medium heat. Add the chives (and garlic, if using) and sauté for 1 to 2 minutes until slightly wilted. Remove from the heat.

2 In a bowl combine the whole eggs, egg whites, Parmesan cheese, salt, and pepper. Whisk to blend well. Stir in the chives and roasted peppers.

3 Heat the skillet over medium-high heat for 30 seconds. Hiding it away from the stove, spray it with olive oil spray. Replace on the burner, reduce the heat to medium, and add the remaining 2 teaspoons oil. Pour in the egg mixture and cook, without stirring, for 2 to 3 minutes until the edges are set and starting to brown. Transfer to the oven and bake for 8 to 10 minutes, or until gently puffed and slightly browned. Cut into wedges and serve with the sliced tomatoes and pumpernickel.

Oatmeal-Barley Cakes

Whole barley is available in health food stores, from Bob's Red Mill Natural Foods, Inc. (see page 70), and from Western Trails, Inc. (800-759-5489 or www.cowboy-foods.com). For these cakes, a 50-50 mixture of Bob's whole hull-less barley and Cowboy's whole grain purple Nu-barley seems to work best.

9½ cups water

1 cup whole hull-less barley

1 cup steel-cut oats, such as McCann's Irish Oatmeal

2 teaspoons kosher salt

2 to 3 tablespoons boiling water, if needed

Canola or olive oil spray

1 To make the cereal, bring the water to a boil in a large nonstick saucepan over high heat. Add the barley and reduce the heat to medium-high. Cook, uncovered, for 50 minutes.

2 Add the oats and salt. Reduce the heat to medium and cook for 15 minutes, stirring occasionally. Reduce the heat to low and continue cooking for 10 to 15 minutes until very thick. Stir often to dislodge any oatmeal that sticks to the bottom of the pan. If the oatmeal cannot be dislodged or becomes too thick to stir, add 2 to 3 tablespoons boiling water. Transfer to a bowl or plastic container and cool to room temperature. Cover and refrigerate until ready to form the cakes.

3 To form the cakes, place a 6 by 12-inch piece of plastic wrap on the counter. Fill a ¼-cup dry measure with cereal and unmold in the center of the plastic by tapping the edge of the cup against it. Fold one end of the plastic over the mound of cereal and press gently to form a 3-inch cake. Fold the other end of the plastic over the cake and set aside. Repeat with the remaining cereal, forming 15 or 16 cakes. (The cakes can be prepared to this point and refrigerated in an airtight container for 1 week.)

4 Heat a large nonstick skillet sprayed with canola or olive oil over medium-high heat. (If you desire more fat, use ¼ teaspoon oil per cake.) Add 5 or 6 cakes and cook, gently flattening them with a pancake turner, for 5 minutes, or until nicely browned. Adjust the heat to pre-

vent scorching. Turn and cook, gently flattening them, for another 5 minutes, or until crisp and nicely browned on the second side. The cakes should now be about 3½ inches in diameter. Use an inverted pancake turner at right angels to the first one to push any stray grains back into the cake. Serve immediately.

Breakfast Leek and Onion "Pizzas"

For variety, substitute other sautéed vegetables (mushrooms, for example) for the onion mixture.

MAKES 3 SERVINGS

> 6 Oatmeal-Barley Cakes (page 72)
> 1½ teaspoons canola or olive oil
> 1 cup thinly sliced onions
> 1 cup thinly sliced leeks
> ½ cup thinly sliced shallots
> Salt and freshly ground black pepper
> 9 ounces sliced part-skim mozzarella or reduced-fat Swiss cheese,
>   cut into ½-inch strips

1 Prepare the oatmeal-barley cakes as directed.

2 Meanwhile, heat the oil in a nonstick skillet over medium heat. Add the onions, leeks, and shallots. Sauté for about 5 minutes until soft. Season generously with salt and pepper.

3 Distribute the vegetables over the oatmeal cakes and top with crossed cheese strips. Cover and cook for 3 minutes, or until the cheese is melted. Serve immediately.

Warm Strawberries Breakfast "Shortcakes"

For a change of pace, pile the warm strawberries on the oatmeal-barley cakes.

MAKES 3 SERVINGS

> 2 pounds firm low-fat tofu
>
> 1 tablespoon canola oil
>
> Salt
>
> 6 Oatmeal-Barley Cakes (page 72)
>
> 3 cups large strawberries, halved lengthwise

1 Preheat the broiler. Drain the tofu and pat dry between 2 kitchen towels. Cut each slab crosswise into 5 pieces. Set aside 1 piece for another use. Remove the grill rack from a nonstick broiler pan. Brush the bottom of the pan with 1½ teaspoons of the oil and arrange the remaining 9 tofu pieces in one layer. Brush with the remaining oil and season lightly with salt. Broil 3 inches from the heat for 5 minutes, or until nicely browned and slightly puffed. Turn and broil for 3 to 5 minutes, or until browned and puffed on the second side. Transfer to a platter and cover loosely with aluminum foil to keep warm.

2 Meanwhile, prepare the oatmeal-barley cakes according to the directions. They should be nicely browned and crisp.

3 Replace the grill rack on the broiler pan and arrange the strawberries on it cut side up. Broil for 1 to 2 minutes until slightly brown at the edges.

4 Place 2 oatmeal cakes, ends touching, on each of 3 plates. Arrange 3 pieces of tofu across the 2 cakes and top with the warm strawberries. Serve immediately.

Scrambled Eggs with Slow-Roasted Tomatoes and Marjoram

Makes 3 servings

3 whole eggs

12 egg whites

Salt and freshly ground black pepper

6 Oatmeal-Barley Cakes (page 72)

1 tablespoon canola or olive oil

1½ cups sliced Slow-Roasted Plum Tomatoes (page 61)

2 teaspoons chopped fresh marjoram

1 Combine the whole eggs and egg whites in a bowl or measuring cup and whisk to blend well. Season with salt and pepper to taste.

2 Prepare the oatmeal-barley cakes according to the recipe. They should be nicely browned and crisp.

3 Meanwhile, heat the oil in a large nonstick skillet over medium heat. Add the eggs and stir them with a wooden spatula, moving the cooked eggs to the surface and the liquid eggs to the bottom of the pan. When they are about three-fourths cooked, distribute the sliced tomatoes and marjoram over them and stir to incorporate. When they are firm but still moist, remove from the heat. Divide the eggs and oatmeal cakes among 3 plates and serve immediately.

Midday Meals

Portobello "Pizzas"

With a green salad, these pizza impersonators make a tasty hot lunch. You can also serve them as an amusing appetizer or side dish in a more elaborate Italian menu. If you have marinara sauce on hand, they involve minimal time and effort.

MAKES 2 TO 3 SERVINGS

2 cups Basic Marinara Sauce (page 63)

Olive oil spray

Eight 6-ounce portobello mushroom caps

1 tablespoon extra virgin olive oil

Salt and freshly ground black pepper

8 ounces shredded part-skim mozzarella

3 tablespoons grated Parmesan cheese

1 Preheat the oven to 450 degrees.

2 Bring the marinara sauce to a boil in a saucepan over medium-high heat and reduce to 1⅓ cups.

> **MUSHROOM FACTS**
>
> Mushrooms have been known to help cleanse the digestive system, as well as boost the immune system. Some mushrooms, including shiitake and enoki, are rich in lentinan, a complex molecule that stimulates the immune system. But mushrooms are also popular because they're extremely low in fat and calories and extremely high in flavor.

3 Spray a nonstick jelly-roll pan or rimmed baking sheet with olive oil spray. Place the mushroom caps, gill side up, on the pan. Brush lightly with the olive oil and season generously with salt and pepper. Spoon 2 to 3 tablespoons reduced marinara sauce into each cap and spread it around. Top with mozzarella and sprinkle with Parmesan cheese. Bake for 10 minutes, or until the mushrooms are tender. Serve immediately.

Warm Lentil Salad
with Spinach and Broiled Salmon

Although any brown lentils will do, the nutty flavor and firm texture of Spanish Pardina lentils makes them ideal for this recipe. They are available from Bob's Red Mill Natural Foods, Inc. (see page 70). Take care to avoid overcooking them.

MAKES 3 SERVINGS

2 tablespoons balsamic vinegar

2 teaspoons Dijon mustard

3 teaspoons extra virgin olive oil

1 cup brown lentils, preferably Spanish Pardina, picked over and rinsed

¼ cup finely chopped shallots

¼ cup minced flat-leaf parsley

¾ teaspoon kosher salt

Freshly ground black pepper

8 cups fresh spinach, washed and stemmed

2 tablespoons Basic Balsamic Vinaigrette (page 65)

1 pound skinless salmon fillet, cut in 3 equal pieces

1   To make the dressing, combine the vinegar, mustard, and 2 teaspoons of the oil in a small measuring cup and whisk to blend.

2   Bring 4 cups water to a boil in a saucepan and add the lentils. Boil gently, uncovered, for 20 minutes until tender but not mushy. Drain well and transfer to a bowl. Add the dressing, shallots, parsley, kosher salt, and pepper to taste. Toss well and cover with aluminum foil to keep warm. (The lentils may be prepared up to 8 hours in advance and refrigerated. Reheat in the microwave before serving.)

3   Meanwhile, place the spinach in a bowl and toss with the Basic Balsamic Vinaigrette.

4 Preheat the broiler. Brush the salmon with the remaining teaspoon oil and season generously on both sides with salt and pepper. Broil the salmon, skin side up, for 4 minutes. Turn and broil for 4 minutes, or until lightly browned and just barely cooked through.

5 To serve, divide the spinach among 3 plates. Spoon the warm lentil salad over the spinach and top with a piece of salmon. Serve immediately.

Hearty Chicken, Mushroom, and Barley Soup

Whole hull-less barley is available in health food stores and from Bob's Red Mill Natural Foods, Inc. (see page 70), and from Western Trails, Inc. (see page 72). Serve with a spinach and red onion salad and Basic Roquefort Dressing (page 64). Follow with fresh fruit for dessert.

MAKES 4 TO 6 SERVINGS

8 to 9 cups chicken broth

½ cup whole hull-less barley

1 cup chopped onions

1 cup chopped carrots

1 teaspoon fresh thyme leaves

½ teaspoon dried sage

1 tablespoon extra virgin olive oil

1 tablespoon minced garlic

1 pound cremini or white mushrooms, sliced ¼ inch thick

Kosher salt

Freshly ground black pepper

1 pound cooked chicken or turkey, diced or shredded

2 tablespoons amontillado sherry, or to taste

3 tablespoons minced flat-leaf parsley

1 Combine 8 cups of the broth, the barley, onions, carrots, thyme, and sage in a large pot or Dutch oven. Bring to a boil. Reduce heat and simmer, covered, for 1 hour.

2 Meanwhile, heat the oil in a large nonstick skillet over medium heat. Add the garlic and sauté for 1 minute. Increase the heat to medium-high, add the mushrooms, and season generously with salt and pepper. Cook, tossing and stirring the mushrooms, until they give up their liquid and most of it has evaporated, about 5 minutes. Set aside.

3 To the broth, add the mushrooms, chicken, 1 teaspoon salt, and black pepper to taste. Simmer, covered, for 20 minutes longer. If the soup is too thick, add the remaining broth and cook for 2 minutes. Stir in the sherry and parsley. Serve immediately.

Green Bean–Tomato Salad with Tuna, Anchovies, and Olives

This salad offers classic niçoise flavors in a low-fat, low-glycemic incarnation. You may substitute other fish, hot or cold, for the tuna in this salad. Salmon, swordfish, and halibut make excellent choices. In a pinch, you may even substitute canned tuna for fresh, but the result will not be quite as luxurious.

MAKES 3 SERVINGS

1½ pounds green beans, trimmed

2 cups sliced Slow-Roasted Plum Tomatoes (page 61), at room temperature

3 tablespoons chopped anchovies

2 tablespoons sliced pitted niçoise olives

1 teaspoon fresh thyme leaves

1 tablespoon minced flat-leaf parsley

Salt and freshly ground black pepper

¾ pound fresh tuna steak, 1 inch thick

1 teaspoon extra virgin olive oil

1 lemon, cut into 6 wedges

4 cups torn arugula

1 Bring a large pot of water to a boil and add the green beans. Cook for 4 minutes from the time they enter the water. Transfer to an ice-water bath to stop the cooking. Drain well and dry between 2 kitchen towels. Transfer to a bowl. Add the tomatoes.

2 Rinse the chopped anchovies under cold running water. Gently pat dry between paper towels.

3 Add the anchovies, olives, thyme, and parsley to the beans. Season with salt and pepper and toss well.

4 Prepare a hot fire in the grill. Brush the tuna on both sides with the oil and season well with salt and pepper. Grill for 3 to 4 minutes per side for medium rare. Cut into 1-inch chunks.

5 Just before serving, squeeze the juice from 3 of the lemon wedges onto the bean salad and toss.

6 To serve, distribute the arugula among 3 plates. Mound the green bean mixture on the arugula and top with the warm tuna chunks. Place 1 lemon wedge on each plate and serve immediately.

Crab Bundles with Avocado-Ginger Sauce

In the absence of tortillas and other flatbreads, lettuce leaves come in handy for wrapping. They're fragile, though, and lead to rather messy meals, so make sure you're among friends when you serve this dish. If you're fastidious, or expect fastidious guests, present this as a composed salad on a bed of romaine. It will be considerably less fun to eat, but just as delicious. The high fat content of avocados has scared away fat-restricting dieters for years. Actually, the monounsaturated fats found in avocados benefit the heart and have no effect on insulin levels. Since crabmeat contains little intrinsic fat, it provides an ideal opportunity for enjoying this luxurious source of healthy fat.

MAKES 4 SERVINGS

1 cup nonfat plain yogurt

1 ripe Hass avocado, peeled and seeded

1 tablespoon brown rice vinegar

1 tablespoon Japanese soy sauce

2 tablespoons minced pickled ginger, drained

½ cup finely chopped red onion

Salt and freshly ground black pepper

16 ounces lump crabmeat, picked over

2 cups finely chopped English cucumbers
  (peeling is optional)

2 cups finely chopped red radishes

2 heads Boston lettuce, leaves separated

1   To make the sauce, combine the yogurt, avo-cado, vinegar, and soy sauce in a food processor. Pulse to a slightly chunky consistency, scraping down the sides as needed. Transfer to a bowl and stir in the pickled ginger and red onion. Blend well. Season to taste with salt and pepper. (The dressing can be made up to 24 hours in advance and refrigerated.)

2   Divide the crabmeat, cucumbers, and radishes among 4 plates. Arrange the lettuce leaves on a platter. Divide the sauce among 4 small bowls. To eat: Take a lettuce leaf or two. Spoon a little sauce onto the center. Add some crab, cucumber, and radish. Top with a little more sauce. Roll and eat.

Cold Chicken and Cauliflower Salad with Grainy Mustard Dressing

This salad can be prepared without the chicken and served as a potato salad surrogate at a picnic or barbecue. It goes beautifully with fish, especially salmon. Serve with a small piece of whole grain bread or follow with fresh fruit for dessert.

MAKES 3 SERVINGS

1 head cauliflower, approximately 2 pounds, cut into 1-inch pieces

½ cup pureed low-fat silken tofu

6 tablespoons nonfat buttermilk

4 tablespoons Hellmann's light mayonnaise

2 tablespoons French grainy mustard, such as Pommery Moutarde de Meaux

2 tablespoons fresh lemon juice

1 tablespoon Dijon mustard

2 teaspoons sherry vinegar

Salt and freshly ground black pepper

8 ounces cooked chicken, cubed

6 cups torn romaine lettuce

3 cups halved cherry tomatoes

2 tablespoons chopped fresh chives

1   Bring a large pot of water to a boil. Add the cauliflower and cook 4 minutes from the time it enters the water. Transfer to an ice-water bath to stop the cooking. Drain well and dry between 2 kitchen towels. Transfer to a bowl. (The cauliflower may be prepared up to 2 days in advance and refrigerated.)

2   To make the dressing, combine the tofu, buttermilk, mayonnaise, grainy mustard, lemon juice, Dijon mustard, vinegar, salt, and pepper to taste in a bowl or measuring cup. Whisk to blend. (The dressing may be prepared up to 3 days in advance and refrigerated.)

3   Add the chicken to the cauliflower. Add approximately half the dressing and toss to coat. Adjust seasoning. Add more dressing if needed.

4   To serve, divide the lettuce among 3 plates. Mound the cauliflower-chicken mixture on top of the lettuce and surround with cherry tomatoes. Garnish with the chives. Pass the extra dressing at the table.

Dinner Dishes

Balsamic Grilled Lamb Chops

Notice that this recipe refers to three different grades of balsamic vinegar. Common balsamic vinegar (technically "imitation" balsamic) is very inexpensive and widely available in supermarkets. "Commercial" balsamic (the moderately priced Fini brand) and artisan-made "tradizionale" (the extravagant Cavalli Tradizionale of Reggio-Emilia) can be found in gourmet shops and specialty food catalogs such as Cook's Wares (800-915-9788 or www.cookswares.com). Cheap balsamic works in the marinade, but not as a finishing sauce. For drizzling over the chops, the commercial grade is satisfactory; the tradizionale is divine.

MAKES 4 SERVINGS

1 cup balsamic vinegar

¼ cup Roasted Garlic Paste (page 62)

¼ cup Dijon mustard

1 tablespoon extra virgin olive oil

1 tablespoon chopped fresh rosemary

1 teaspoon kosher salt

1 teaspoon freshly ground black pepper

Eight 4½-ounce bone-in loin or rib lamb chops, trimmed of all visible fat

1 tablespoon high-quality commercial (such as Fini brand) or artisan-made balsamic vinegar "tradizionale" (optional)

1 To make the marinade, combine the vinegar, garlic paste, mustard, and oil in a blender and emulsify. Transfer to a bowl or measuring cup. Stir in the rosemary, salt, and pepper. (The marinade may be prepared up to 2 days in advance and refrigerated.)

2 Place the chops in a gallon-size heavy-duty Ziploc bag and pour the marinade over them. Turn to coat well. Marinate 1 hour at room temperature or up to 12 hours in the refrigerator.

3 Prepare a hot fire in the grill. Discard the marinade. Grill the chops 4 to 5 minutes per side to medium-rare. Serve immediately, drizzled with the artisan-made vinegar, if desired.

ROASTED SALMON WITH FRESH HERBS AND BROCCOLI RABE WITH ROASTED PEPPERS AND TOMATOES

The salmon in this dinner menu is so easy to prepare that it leaves time for a more involved vegetable accompaniment. The broccoli rabe recipe calls for slow-roasted tomatoes, which can be made well in advance. If you roast the peppers and blanch the broccoli ahead also, this sumptuous meal requires less than 15 minutes. However, if advance preparation does not suit you, serve the salmon with Roasted Garlic Asparagus (page 88) and a tomato salad with Basic Roquefort Dressing (page 64).

Roasted Salmon with Fresh Herbs

Salmon is one of the healthiest dishes you can serve, and even a simple recipe like this can be delicious. It's a great meal to serve to guests.

MAKES 4 SERVINGS

> 1½ teaspoons extra virgin olive oil
> 1¼ pounds skinless salmon fillets
> Salt and freshly ground black pepper
> 2 to 3 tablespoons chopped fresh herbs (parsley, rosemary, and thyme; or parsley, tarragon, and chives)

1 Preheat the oven to 450 degrees. Brush a baking dish with ½ teaspoon of the olive oil and add the salmon. Brush the salmon with the remaining 1 teaspoon oil and season generously with salt and pepper.

2 Roast for 8 to 12 minutes until just cooked through. Remove from the oven and sprinkle with the herbs. Serve hot, warm, or at room temperature.

Broccoli Rabe with Roasted Peppers and Tomatoes

2 red bell peppers

2 yellow bell peppers

2 bunches broccoli rabe, about 2 pounds

1 tablespoon plus 1 teaspoon kosher salt

1 tablespoon extra virgin olive oil

1 tablespoon minced garlic

¼ teaspoon hot red pepper flakes

2 cups thickly sliced Slow-Roasted Plum Tomatoes (page 61)

Freshly ground black pepper

1 Roast the bell peppers by thoroughly charring the skins under the broiler. Transfer to a paper bag and allow to steam for 10 to 15 minutes to loosen the skins. Remove the stems, skins, seeds, and membranes. Cut the flesh into ½-inch dice and set aside with any collected juice. (The peppers may be prepared to this point up to 3 days in advance and refrigerated.)

2 Bring a large pot of water to a boil. Add the broccoli rabe and 1 tablespoon salt. Cook 3 minutes and transfer immediately to an ice-water bath to stop the cooking. Drain and dry between 2 kitchen towels. Roll up the towels and squeeze gently to remove any excess water. Set aside. (The broccoli rabe may be prepared to this point up to 3 days in advance and refrigerated.)

3 Heat the oil in a large deep nonstick skillet over medium heat. Add the garlic and red pepper flakes. Sauté for 1 minute. Add the roasted bell peppers, broccoli rabe, the remaining salt, the roasted tomatoes, and black pepper to taste. Cook, tossing frequently, for 2 to 3 minutes, or until heated through. Serve immediately.

Shrimp Marinara with Garlic Asparagus

Timing is everything in this meal. While your oven is warming, peel and devein the shrimp and then peel the asparagus (see page 88). Proceed through step 2 of the shrimp recipe. Then toss the asparagus in Roasted Garlic Paste (page 62), season with salt, and pop them in the oven. Finish the shrimp and remove the asparagus from the oven. Follow with fresh fruit for dessert.

MAKES 4 SERVINGS

2 teaspoons extra virgin olive oil

1 tablespoon minced garlic

3 tablespoons minced flat-leaf parsley

1¼ pounds large shrimp, peeled and deveined

Salt and freshly ground black pepper

¼ cup bottled clam juice or homemade shrimp broth

2 cups Basic Marinara Sauce (page 63)

1 teaspoon anchovy paste

1 Heat the oil in a large nonstick skillet over medium heat. Add the garlic and 1 tablespoon of the parsley. Sauté for 1 minute. Add the shrimp and season generously with salt and pepper. Cook, turning frequently, for about 2 minutes. Add the clam juice and cook for 1 minute, turning the shrimp. They should still be slightly underdone at this point—not fully opaque. Using a slotted spoon, remove the shrimp to a sieve over a bowl. Pour any liquid back into the skillet.

2 Add the marinara sauce and anchovy paste to the skillet. Stir to blend. Bring to a simmer and cook, stirring frequently, for 5 to 10 minutes until the sauce is thick, with almost no watery liquid visible.

3 Return the shrimp to the skillet and cook for 1 to 2 minutes until opaque and heated through. Do not overcook. Serve immediately, garnished with the remaining parsley.

Roasted Garlic Asparagus

You may not relish peeling your asparagus, but if you force yourself to do it, you'll love the results. Peeled asparagus cook evenly and become silky, sweet, and wholly edible. In response to an instruction in one of Julia Child's books, I peeled them once and have not been able to eat them any other way since. Be sure to salt them before roasting. To keep raw asparagus fresh in the refrigerator, trim the stem ends and stand them upright in about ½ inch of water. Loosely drape a plastic bag over the tips.

MAKES 6 SERVINGS

> 3 pounds fresh asparagus, stems peeled
> 1 tablespoon Roasted Garlic Paste (page 62)
> Salt

1 Preheat the oven to 450 degrees. Lay the asparagus flat on a nonstick jelly-roll pan. (Do not crowd the asparagus. If they do not all fit in a single layer on one pan, plan to roast the asparagus in two batches, dividing the paste between them.) Drizzle with roasted garlic paste and toss well to coat. Salt generously.

2 Roast for 5 to 8 minutes, depending on the thickness of the spears, until crisp-tender. Serve immediately.

SMOTHERED PORK TENDERLOIN WITH VIDALIA ONIONS AND GRAPES WITH TURNIP GRATIN WITH GARLIC AND THYME

Notice that the pork and turnip recipes require slightly different oven temperatures. First preheat the oven to 400 degrees and prepare the turnip gratin. Remove from the oven after 15 minutes instead of 20. Increase the oven temperature to 450 degrees. Proceed with the pork. When the pork reaches an internal temperature of 150 degrees, transfer it to a platter and turn the oven temperature down to 350 degrees and immediately slide in the gratin. Bake for 5 to 10 minutes while the pork rests and you prepare the sauce. Alternatively, you could fully cook the gratin ahead of time and then reheat it in the microwave.

Smothered Pork Tenderloin with Vidalia Onions and Grapes

Carefully trimmed cooked pork tenderloin contains only 1.3 grams of fat per ounce. So as you trim, be thorough in your work and do not be distressed by the small amount of meat lost along with the fat. This waste is small compared to the human loss associated with excess saturated fat consumption. Also, be sure you do not overcook your lean little tenderloin. If you're careful, it will live up to its name, but it can also turn tough and dry in a hurry.

MAKES 4 SERVINGS

1¼ pounds pork tenderloin, visible fat removed

Salt and freshly ground black pepper

1 teaspoon extra virgin olive oil

½ cup sliced Vidalia onion

1½ cups grapes (preferably Concord)

1 tablespoon balsamic vinegar

1   Preheat the oven to 450 degrees. Season the pork generously with salt and pepper. Heat the oil in a cast-iron skillet over medium-high heat and add the pork. (If necessary, cut the pork into 2 pieces to fit the skillet.) Brown the pork on all sides and transfer to the oven.

2   For slightly pink meat, roast for approximately 10 minutes, to an internal temperature of 150 degrees on an instant-read thermometer inserted into the thickest portion of the meat. Transfer the meat to a platter and allow to rest for 5 to 10 minutes. (The internal temperature of the meat will continue to rise.)

3   Meanwhile, place the skillet over medium heat and add the onion. Cook, stirring frequently, until it begins to soften and brown. Add the grapes and continue cooking for 2 to 3 minutes until the first few grapes split. Stir in the vinegar and any accumulated meat juices. Remove from the heat and adjust the seasoning.

4   Thickly slice the pork on the diagonal and smother with the grape-and-onion mixture. Serve immediately.

Turnip Gratin with Garlic and Thyme

MAKES 4 SERVINGS

2½ pounds purple-top turnips, peeled and sliced ¼ inch thick

Olive or canola oil spray

Salt and freshly ground black pepper

2 teaspoons extra virgin olive oil, canola oil, or butter

2 tablespoons chickpea flour

1½ cups skim milk

1 teaspoon minced garlic

1 teaspoon fresh thyme leaves

1 teaspoon kosher salt

½ cup pureed low-fat silken tofu

1 ounce Gruyère cheese, grated (about 1 cup)

1   Bring a large pot of water to boil. Add the turnips and cook for 4 minutes. (Start counting from the moment you add them.) Transfer to an ice-water bath to stop the cooking. Drain and dry between layers of kitchen towels. (The turnips may be prepared to this point up to 3 days in advance and refrigerated.)

2   Set the rack in the upper third of the oven and preheat to 400 degrees. Spray a 2½-quart baking dish with olive oil spray. Place half the turnips in the dish so that they overlap and lie flat. Season generously with salt and pepper. Add the remaining turnips and season well with salt and pepper.

3   Heat the oil in a saucepan over medium heat. Add the flour and cook, whisking constantly, for 30 seconds. Remove from the heat and vigorously whisk in the milk, dissolving any lumps. Bring the milk to a boil over medium-high heat. Add the garlic, thyme, kosher salt, and pepper to taste. Reduce the heat and simmer for 5 minutes, whisking occasionally. Remove from the heat and whisk in the tofu. Blend well.

4   Pour the sauce over the turnips and sprinkle with the cheese. Bake for 20 minutes until lightly browned and bubbling. (If you are roasting the pork in the same oven, follow the special instructions in the headnote.) Allow to cool 5 minutes before serving.

SPICED TURKEY KEBABS WITH CURRIED SLAW WITH FRUIT AND PISTACHIOS

This menu provides an aromatic and satisfying meal requiring very little effort.

Spiced Turkey Kebabs

During the summer, many local markets offer "London broil–style" turkey—half a boneless skinless breast in the form of a thick steak. One great way to serve it is to marinate it overnight in Indian spices and grill it the next day. The meat can be skewered with or without the usual shish-kebab companions (peppers, onions, cherry tomatoes). The recipe provides plenty of extra spice mixture to use with chicken, duck, lamb, and pork. Store the excess in an airtight container in a cool, dark place and use it as needed. It should keep for up to 6 months.

MAKES 4 SERVINGS

  1 tablespoon ground cumin
  1 tablespoon ground coriander
  1 tablespoon turmeric
  ½ to 1 teaspoon cayenne pepper
  1 tablespoon salt
  1 teaspoon freshly ground black pepper
  1 tablespoon peanut or canola oil
  1 tablespoon minced garlic
  1 tablespoon minced fresh ginger
  2 tablespoons minced onion
  1⅓ pounds boneless skinless turkey breast, cut in 1½-inch chunks

1 To make the spice mix, combine the cumin, coriander, turmeric, cayenne, salt, and pepper in a small nonstick skillet over medium heat. Cook, stirring, for 2 to 3 minutes until

fragrant. Remove from the heat and set aside to cool. Measure out 2 teaspoons (or more to taste) into a medium-sized bowl. Reserve the extra for another use.

2   Add the oil, garlic, ginger, and onion to the spice mix. Whisk to blend. Add the turkey chunks and toss well to coat. (The turkey can be set aside in the refrigerator for up to 24 hours at this point.)

3   Preheat the broiler or prepare a hot fire in the grill. Thread the turkey chunks loosely on the skewers. Broil or grill 4 inches from the heat for about 4 minutes. Turn and broil or grill for approximately 4 minutes longer, or until the turkey is cooked through but not dry. Serve immediately.

Curried Slaw with Fruit and Pistachios

Fresh fruit, cooked or raw, can take the place of chutney as a sweet accompaniment to meats. This slaw goes beautifully with spiced turkey kebabs and other dishes with an Indian flair. It also complements plain grilled pork and duck. The dressing is excellent with crudités, salads, and cold steamed vegetables, as well as poached chicken or fish.

MAKES 6 SERVINGS

½ cup fresh orange juice
½ cup nonfat plain yogurt
2 tablespoons low-fat mayonnaise
1 teaspoon grated orange zest
1 tablespoon chopped fresh mint
1 teaspoon curry powder
½ teaspoon salt or to taste
4 cups finely shredded green cabbage
¼ cup thinly sliced red onion
½ cup halved red grapes
¾ cup peeled, diced apple tossed with 1 teaspoon lemon juice
¼ cup shelled dry-roasted salted pistachios
Freshly ground black pepper

1 To make the dressing, bring the orange juice to a boil in a small saucepan. Reduce to a volume of 2 tablespoons. Remove from the heat and cool to room temperature. Reserve 1½ teaspoons. Set aside the remainder for another use.

2 Combine the orange syrup with the yogurt, mayonnaise, orange zest, mint, curry powder, and salt. Whisk to blend.

3 In a large bowl, combine the cabbage, onion, grapes, apple, and pistachios. Add the dressing and toss well to coat. Add salt and pepper to taste and serve immediately.

Fragrant Lentils with Fennel

MAKES 4 SERVINGS

¾ cup dried brown lentils, preferably Spanish Pardina

1 tablespoon extra virgin olive oil

½ cup chopped fennel

1 teaspoon minced fresh ginger

½ teaspoon ground cumin

½ teaspoon ground coriander

¼ teaspoon ground turmeric

¼ teaspoon ground cinnamon

2 cups water

¾ teaspoon kosher salt

2 tablespoons minced flat-leaf parsley or cilantro

Pinch cayenne pepper

Freshly ground black pepper

1 Pick over lentils to remove any stones. Place in a sieve and rinse under cold running water. Drain and set aside.

2 Heat the oil in a nonstick saucepan over medium heat. Add the fennel, ginger, cumin, coriander, turmeric, and cinnamon. Sauté, stirring often, for 3 minutes, or until the fennel is tender. Add the lentils and stir to coat. Add the water, increase the heat to medium-high, and bring to a boil. Boil gently, uncovered, for 20 minutes, or until the lentils are tender and most of the liquid has evaporated. Stir in the salt, parsley or cilantro, cayenne, and black pepper. Serve immediately.

FILETS MIGNONS WITH SHALLOTS AND GARLIC WITH CREAMY ZUCCHINI PUDDING

This menu provides real comfort food: a warm, creamy vegetable pudding. Classic versions are topped with high-glycemic bread crumbs and laden with heart-unhealthy saturated fat. In this incarnation, low-fat tofu replaces heavy cream and a single egg contributes body and richness. Fresh thyme and a sprinkling of Pecorino Romano cheese complement the delicate flavor of the zucchini without obscuring it. For a pleasant variation, substitute fresh marjoram for thyme and Parmesan cheese for the Pecorino. Although the pudding is paired here with filets mignons, it goes beautifully with almost any grilled or roasted meat, fowl, or fish.

If the same oven is used for the beef and the pudding, prepare the pudding first and remove it from the oven after 20 minutes. When the meat is cooked to the desired doneness, transfer it to a platter and turn the oven temperature down to 400 degrees. Slide the pudding back into the oven for 5 minutes while the beef rests. Alternatively, you could fully cook the pudding ahead of time and reheat it in the microwave.

> **FILET FACTS** Filet mignon is a tender round of steak cut from the thick end of a beef tenderloin. It is the leanest and most tender cut available (which explains its relatively high cost). If it is cooked right, you should be able to cut it with a fork.

Filets Mignons with Shallots and Garlic

Meticulously trimmed beef tenderloin contains just under 3 grams of fat per ounce, about one-third of which is saturated. While a chicken breast contains significantly less fat, beef supplies four times as much iron, so enjoying beef on occasion is completely justified.

MAKES 4 SERVINGS

1 pound filets mignons, 1½ to 2 inches thick, visible fat removed
Salt and freshly ground black pepper
1 teaspoon extra virgin olive oil or porcini mushroom oil

SAUCE

1 tablespoon minced shallots
1 teaspoon minced garlic
1 tablespoon balsamic or sherry vinegar
¼ cup water or fat-free beef broth
Salt and freshly ground black pepper

1   Set the rack in the upper third of the oven and preheat to 500 degrees. Place a cast-iron skillet in the oven for 5 minutes. Season the beef generously with salt and pepper, brush on both sides with the oil, and place in the hot skillet. Roast for 12 to 15 minutes, or until an instant-read thermometer inserted into the thickest part of the meat reads 120 degrees for rare, 125 to 130 degrees for medium-rare, or 135 to 140 degrees for medium. Transfer the meat to a cutting board and allow to rest for 5 minutes. (The temperature of the meat will continue to rise.)

2   To make the sauce, place the skillet over low heat. Add the shallots, garlic, vinegar, water, salt, and pepper to taste, and any collected meat juices. Simmer, scraping up the brown bits, for about 2 minutes, until the garlic and shallots are tender. Remove from the heat.

3   Thickly slice the beef on the diagonal, distribute among 4 plates, and drizzle 1 tablespoon of the sauce on each portion. Serve immediately, passing the extra sauce at the table.

Creamy Zucchini Pudding

MAKES 4 SERVINGS

6 medium zucchini, about 2½ pounds

2½ teaspoons kosher salt

3 teaspoons extra virgin olive oil

1 cup chopped onion

1 tablespoon minced garlic

1 large whole egg

1 cup pureed low-fat silken tofu

1 teaspoon fresh thyme leaves

Freshly ground black pepper

Olive oil spray

2 tablespoons grated Pecorino Romano cheese

1 Set the rack in the upper third of the oven and preheat to 400 degrees.

2 Grate the zucchini in a food processor fitted with a coarse grating disk. Transfer the zucchini to a colander and toss with 2 teaspoons of the salt. Set the colander over a bowl and allow to drain for about 30 minutes. Spread out a kitchen towel and cover with a layer of paper towels. Spread the grated zucchini in a thin layer on the paper towels. Cover with another layer of paper towels and another kitchen towel. Starting at one end, roll up the towels and gently squeeze to remove excess water. Transfer the zucchini to a bowl.

3 Heat 2 teaspoons of the oil in a nonstick skillet over medium heat and add the onion. Sauté for 5 to 7 minutes until soft. Add the garlic and sauté for 1 minute. Remove from the heat and allow to cool for 5 minutes.

4 Lightly beat the egg in a bowl or measuring cup. Add the tofu and the remaining ½ teaspoon salt. Whisk to blend. Add to the zucchini along with the onion mixture, thyme, and black pepper. Stir gently with a fork to combine.

5 Spray a 1½-quart baking dish with olive oil. Spread the zucchini mixture evenly in the dish and smooth it out on top. Sprinkle with the Pecorino and drizzle with the remaining 1 teaspoon oil.

6 Bake for 20 to 25 minutes until lightly browned and bubbling. Serve immediately.

Moroccan Chicken Thighs with Roasted Eggplant

This fragrant chicken stew illustrates one of the many uses of roasted eggplant. Since the eggplant simmers in the sauce for 10 minutes, roast it until it is tender but not soft or it will disintegrate during the final cooking. You can leave the skin on or you can peel it if you wish before cutting it into cubes. If you do not have roasted eggplant, zucchini cut into 1-inch chunks will cook in the allotted time. The stew is excellent (perhaps even better) reheated the next day. Accompany with a green salad and follow with fresh fruit for dessert.

MAKES 4 SERVINGS

8 bone-in chicken thighs, skin and visible fat removed
Salt and freshly ground black pepper
1 tablespoon extra virgin olive oil
1 cup chopped onion
1 tablespoon minced fresh ginger
1 tablespoon minced garlic
1 cinnamon stick
1 teaspoon ground cumin
1 cup diced canned tomatoes, drained
1½ cups chicken broth
1 cup cooked and drained chickpeas
1 cup cubed Roasted Eggplant (page 99)
2 tablespoons minced flat-leaf parsley

1 Season the chicken generously with salt and pepper. Heat the oil in a large nonstick skillet or Dutch oven over medium-high heat. Add the chicken and brown well on both sides, then remove from the skillet.

2 Reduce the heat to medium. Add the onion and sauté, stirring, until soft, about 3 minutes. Add the ginger, garlic, cinnamon stick, and cumin. Cook, stirring, for 1 minute.

Add the tomatoes, broth, and salt and pepper to taste. Return the chicken with any accumulated juices to the pan. Baste with the sauce. Cover and simmer for 15 minutes. Add the chickpeas and roasted eggplant, and simmer for 10 minutes.

3   Adjust the seasoning and remove the cinnamon stick. Garnish with the parsley. Serve immediately.

Roasted Eggplant

MAKES 6 CUPS

> 2 pounds eggplants, ends trimmed and halved lengthwise
> Salt and freshly ground black pepper (optional)
> 1 teaspoon extra virgin olive oil

1   Preheat the oven to 450 degrees. Using a two-tined carving fork, pierce the cut sides of the eggplants all over, down to but not through the skin. Season with salt and pepper, if desired. Brush a nonstick baking sheet with the oil and place the eggplants cut side down.

2   Roast long, narrow Asian eggplants and Italian baby eggplants for 10 to 15 minutes, or until tender; roast Western globe or purple eggplants for 20 to 30 minutes, or until tender. If the eggplants will be cooked further in another recipe, remove from the oven when they yield to a fork but are not completely soft.

3   Peel the eggplants, if desired. Slice or cut into cubes and adjust the seasoning. Serve warm or at room temperature, or store in the refrigerator for up to 1 week.

Buffalo Chili

A first-rate nutritional profile makes buffalo a heart-healthy choice for red meat lovers. It contains one-sixth the total fat and one-sixth the saturated fat of "lean only" beef tenderloin. It also contains 30 percent less cholesterol. Happily, buffalo has become increasingly available over the past few years. It tastes just like beef in this savory chili. Serve it with a green salad dressed with balsamic vinaigrette.

MAKES 4 SERVINGS

1 tablespoon extra virgin olive oil

1 cup chopped onion

½ cup chopped green bell pepper

1 tablespoon minced garlic

One 4-ounce can mild green chiles, drained, seeded, and chopped

¼ cup chili powder

1 tablespoon unsweetened cocoa

1½ teaspoons ground cumin

1½ teaspoons dried oregano

½ teaspoon ground allspice

1 pound ground buffalo

1 cup cooked or canned kidney beans, drained

One 28-ounce can crushed tomatoes with added puree

⅔ cup beef broth

2 teaspoons kosher salt

Freshly ground black pepper

4 tablespoons low-fat sour cream (optional)

4 tablespoons sliced scallions (optional)

1 Heat the oil in a large nonstick skillet over medium heat. Add the onion, green pepper, and garlic. Cook for 5 minutes, or until soft. Add the chiles, chili powder, cocoa, cumin, oregano, and allspice. Cook for 1 minute, stirring constantly.

2 Add the buffalo and cook, breaking up the meat, for 7 minutes, or until brown. Add the beans, tomatoes, broth, salt, and pepper. Bring to a boil. Reduce the heat to low, cover, and simmer, stirring occasionally, for 25 to 30 minutes until thick. Serve immediately, garnished with a dollop of sour cream and a sprinkling of scallions, if desired.

Not a Cook? Not a Problem

Don't feel you have to be a gourmet cook if you want to be healthy. There are many ways to eat well without spending a lot of time in the kitchen.

Many supermarkets these days have gourmet and/or health food sections, where you can pick up ready-made meals (or portions thereof). For instance, mesclun salad in bags, prewashed chopped vegetables, couscous and grilled vegetables, organic nuts and dried berries.

Here are some other quick-and-easy meal suggestions:

Breakfast

- My favorite: one or two hard-boiled eggs, one can of sardines (packed in oil), salad greens with chickpeas, topped with balsamic vinegar.

- Grilled salmon, tomato and onion salad with olive oil and vinegar.

- Low-fat yogurt with nuts and fresh berries.

- Slow-cooked oatmeal with sliced apples and/or berries and cinnamon.

Lunch

- Grilled tuna with arugula and a tossed green salad with oil and vinegar dressing.

- Green salad with a variety of lettuces and sprouts, tomatoes, mushrooms, and onions, topped with grilled chicken and mustard dressing.

- Cottage cheese with mixed berries or melon slices.

Dinner

- Turkey burgers. Make like hamburgers, using ground turkey instead. Serve with grilled or steamed vegetables.

- Salmon salad. Mix a quarter pound of fresh salmon or canned salmon with chopped carrots, chopped scallions, and sprouts. Add olive oil and balsamic vinegar or a tablespoon of low-fat mayonnaise.

Don't be afraid to mix and match. There's no reason you can't have a turkey burger for breakfast or an omelet for dinner. And whatever you do, don't get stuck on perfection. Make room in your life for recreational eating. If, on occasion, you want to go out and enjoy a traditional Italian pasta meal, or a rice-heavy Cuban dinner, go right ahead. If you keep the Paleotech Diet principles in mind at least 80 percent of the time, you'll be in great shape.

4 High-Tech Secrets of Weight Control

Seven steps to burning fat

As we now know, the unfortunate truth is that the human body is not cut out for the twenty-first century. Why? Because underneath all our modern trappings and scientific advancements lurk the hormones of cavemen. The differences in their lifestyle and ours have, in many ways, led to a greatly improved quality of life for human beings. In other ways, however, these differences have led to the incredible hormonal imbalances that have created the current epidemic in obesity.

If current statistics are correct, 63 percent of all Americans are overweight, with about fifty million on diets at any given time, and a substantial number of the overweight are obese (that's means they're 20 percent over their ideal body weight). In an article in the *New York Times* titled "95% Regain Lost Weight. Or Do They?" (May 25, 1999), Professor James Hill of the University of Colorado, referred to as the dean of American obesity studies, said, "Becoming obese is a normal response to the American environment." The Centers for Disease Control calls obesity an epidemic, and notes that the top ten causes of death due to diseases are attributable to health risks associated with excess body fat.

So with fifty million of us (and that's only in America) on diets at any one time, you'd think that the subject of weight control would be nailed by now. You'd think that if you have or had a problem with weight, the whole range of available information, diets, diet books, plans, gadgets, and programs would have set you free long ago. Obviously, that hasn't happened. And the reason is that we've been approaching the problem from the wrong perspective.

Feel the Burn

What do you think about when you think about losing weight? Exercise? Calories? Fat? Carbohydrates? *Hormones?* No one ever thinks about hormones; yet hormones are what control how and when we *burn fat,* and that controls how and when we lose weight. If you're not thinking in terms of hormones, you will lose water weight, muscle tone, and even pounds—and then gain them all back again.

Your Healthy High-Tech Body goal is not so much to lose weight as to burn fat and fuel more efficiently, to get your hormones working at peak capacity. The by-product of that is reaching a healthy weight for your body, working within your body's guidelines.

In order to achieve that goal, all systems must be working together to keep your hormones in balance. That means you *cannot lose weight just by dieting alone.* You have to add in exercise, because it affects your hormones. You have to get enough sleep and avoid stress, because both affect your hormones. And, because you may have to bring some imbalanced hormones back into alignment, you may have to take some hormone-influencing supplements.

As a nation, we are hormonally out of whack. This problem can't be fixed by concentrating on diet alone. Following the Paleotech Diet is a great start. But just because you get one hormonal component in order doesn't mean your whole system will function at its best.

WORLDWATCH NEWS RELEASE, MARCH 2000

For the first time in human history the number of overweight people rivals the number of underweight people, according to a new report from the Worldwatch Institute, a Washington, D.C.–based research organization. While the world's underfed population has declined slightly since 1980 to 1.1 billion, the number of overweight people has surged to 1.1 billion.

What can we do? We can't go back to a Paleolithic lifestyle to get healthy. That's why we need High-Tech solutions. High Tech doesn't necessarily mean technology based. It means looking at health with the full twenty-first-century understanding of how the body works.

Toward Healthy Leanness

How can we be so sure that the epidemic of obesity isn't just due to an overabundance of food and an underwhelming amount of discipline? Because more than 90 percent of dieters gain back every pound they lose. It can't be true that all those millions and millions of people are simply not trying hard enough.

Once again, we have to go back to our ancestry and the fact that as animals we have been shaped through evolutionary design to respond to food in a number of ways—mainly to eat as much as possible when food is available as a means of storing energy (in the form of fat) to protect us against potential lean periods and famines. It is a powerful anticipatory response controlled by molecular messengers, hormones, and chemicals that tell us to eat, to stop eating, to gain or lose weight.

The chemical messengers controlling weight and appetite are produced in a part of the brain called the hypothalamus, which has been called a biological thermostat. The size of an almond, this tiny body part regulates body temperature, blood pressure, and heartbeat, as well as the metabolism of fats and carbohydrates.

When the system of chemical messengers controlling weight and appetite is operating properly, it will keep you within a certain weight range, called a **setpoint**, a feature, mostly inherited, that varies about 10 percent from your midpoint weight. The setpoint of a 180-pound man, for example, might range from 162 to 198. The setpoint theory was proposed by William Bennet and Joel Gurin in their book *The Dieter's Dilemma: Eating Less & Weighing More*. Bennet and Gurin were the first to say, based on careful analysis, that there is a control system built into every person dictating how much he or she will weigh. Since then scientists have continued to identify genes, brain chemicals, and hormones that influence that dictation. Bennet and Gurin believed that managing weight meant a lot more than just measuring calories on a balance sheet, and they were the first to debunk the notion that a problem in controlling weight was simply a matter of behavioral weakness and lack of willpower.

However, the "dieter's dilemma" keeps getting worse as we continue to damage our weight control system and disrupt its ability to perform through our mega-portion diets, lack of fitness, and general misunderstanding of weight management. This disruption is aggravated by the battle between our Paleolithic metabolism and our modern appetites for the oceans of available foods, especially those super-engorged with fats, sugars, and carbs.

The supersize meal at McDonald's, for instance, packs a whopping 1,340 calories for a Coke, cheeseburger, and fries. Originally, McDonald's offered only one size portion of french fries, and that contained about 200 calories. By the year 2000, the supersize portion of fries had ballooned to 610 calories. And that's just one example of the dietary warfare being waged against our bodies by food industries that are spending $40 billion a year on advertising designed to neutralize our ability to restrain ourselves.

A study at the City University of New York, published in the *American Journal of Clinical Nutrition* (October 2000), showed that one-third of American adults get almost half of their calories from high-calorie, low-nutrient foods like candy, chips, soda, and ice cream. And it also showed that most of the time, these foods were eaten not in addition to, but instead of, healthy foods.

The bottom line is that the food and dietary landscape we inhabit is hostile to our well-being. Our ability to control ourselves in the face of this is beyond what we are capable of, biologically and behaviorally. We're constantly consuming "heart attacks on plates" as less of the food we eat is intended to impart health and instead our meals alter the very fabric of our biology, blowing the top lid off our setpoints, making us fat, and laying down the foundations for high blood pressure, glucose toxicity, adult-onset diabetes, cancers, stroke, and heart disease.

Throughout your life, you'll slide up and down your setpoint range, based on a *complex group of dynamics*, including hereditary factors, hormone levels, environment, gender, age, eating habits, fitness levels, and brain chemicals like leptin.

In 1994, Dr. Jeffrey Friedman of Rockefeller University in New York discovered a small protein, produced by fat cells, that acts like a hormone, signaling the brain to tell the body when to eat. He called it leptin. The theory was that the brain responds to leptin deficiencies by telling the body to eat, eat, and eat more. It seemed that obesity might be caused by leptin deficiencies and could be treated by supplying the body with this hormonelike substance. Unfortunately, studies showed that this theory did not hold up.

Scientists now know that overweight people have plenty of leptin, although they become resistant to it the same way a diabetic becomes resistant to insulin. Scientists also know that when you diet and lose weight, you make less leptin. Then the brain signals the body to eat more, increasing leptin levels again. Some new studies, however, have shown that leptin can be effective when combined with other existing diet drugs.

In an article titled "How the Body Knows When to Gain or Lose" (*New York Times*, October 17, 2000), writer Gina Kolata notes that scientists are now finding dozens of molecules in the brain that may lead to new treatments for obesity, and that "all the new research points to the conclusion that obesity is a hormonal problem resulting from too little or too much of molecules like leptin . . . that signal the body to eat or abstain." If scientists can discover the particular hormone(s) that is causing the problem, they may be able to find that magic pill we've all been looking for.

The search for that magic pill is ongoing. There is an ever-increasing number of theories as to why we gain weight and have such difficulties losing it, and there is an equally growing number of studies to prove each one of these theories:

- For instance, scientists have discovered an injectable drug called Axokine that appears to reset the brain's setpoint, making a lower weight seem natural. Axokine lets the body bypass its leptin resistance. Instead, it mimics the appetite-suppressant qualities of cytokines, the hormones that are released into your body whenever you're ill or injured.

- Another study involved genetically engineered mice that were able to dramatically increase fat-burning capabilities. Scientists created mice that lacked an enzyme involved in fat metabolism, known as ACC2. Those mice had 50 percent less body fat than normal mice because they continually burned fatty acids. So they could eat much more food than other mice and still weighed 15 to 20 percent less. Scientists are searching for a pill that could be used to block the ACC2 enzyme in humans.

- There's another enzyme called fatty acid synthase that is involved in telling the brain that it's hungry. Researchers at Johns Hopkins Medical Institute discovered a synthetic compound called C75 that seems to inhibit fatty acid synthase, thereby tricking the brain into thinking it's not hungry.

- Researchers from the Whitehead Institute and Genset Corporation have found a new compound called gAcrp30 that controls weight gain in obese mice without affecting their food intake. Administered daily, it caused the mice to lose weight, even though they were eating large meals high in fat and sugar. Much more research is needed to determine whether this substance can be used in humans.

- And then there's the virus theory. Scientists found that both mice and chicken infected with a common human virus, adenovirus-36, had much more fat than uninfected animals. When they tested overweight humans, they found that 20 to 30 percent of them were infected with the virus, compared to about 5 percent of the lean population. The theory here is that the virus somehow increased the number of fat cells in those who were infected. Researchers are working toward finding an antiviral medication or vaccine that would eliminate this virus and decrease fat cells.

- Another study found that marijuanalike substances, called endocannabinoids, in the brain stimulate appetite. Mice that had been genetically altered so that they could not respond to endocannabinoids ate less than normal mice, and when normal mice were given substances that block endocannabinoids, they also ate less than normal. The study also found that endocannabinoids are part of the complex brain systems controlled by leptin. However, scientists still have no idea how endocannabinoids are created by the body, or exactly how they work. Dr. Rudy Leibel, head of molecular genetics at Columbia University, told the *New York Times* (April 11, 2001) that the study "suggests that it will probably not be possible to deliver, in a pharmaceutical sense, a single magic bullet or knockout punch against these systems in the brain, since they are so highly redundant and backed up."

In all of these early studies, proving the theory is easier than finding the "cure." Some of the drugs produce unpleasant side effects, and their long-term results are unknown. But all these studies are helping scientists discover the so-far illusive mechanisms of weight control and will hopefully lead to some practical answers within the near future.

And, since all of the studies are still in early stages, you'll have to look elsewhere for the time being if you want to burn fat and reach your weight goals. The Healthy High-Tech Body goal is not only to lose weight and get to the low end of your setpoint range, but to get there looking great, having adequate muscle mass, and a respectably reduced percentage of body fat. In order to do that, you need to follow the seven steps to burning fat.

The Seven Steps to Burning Fat

A Healthy High-Tech Body then is one that embraces *healthy leanness*, where the fat on and in your body isn't killing you. If you want to achieve healthy leanness, there are seven steps you need to take, essential to fat burning and lean muscle building:

> **THE WINNING FORMULA IS A COMBINATION OF:**
> Aerobic exercise
> Anaerobic exercise
> Prudent eating

1 Eat according to Paleotech Diet guidelines.

2 Change toxic eating habits.

3 Control insulin, glucagon, and cortisol so that you don't accumulate fat around your waistline and stomach, *anywhere you don't want it.*

4 Exercise *aerobically* to enhance long-term fat burning.

5 Exercise *anaerobically* to build and increase fat-burning muscle.

6 Get enough sleep, about eight hours, and control stress.

7 Take the right nutraceuticals or drugs to improve metabolic performance, balance brain chemistry, and control hormones.

Steps 1 to 3: Healthy Eating

Hopefully, you have already begun to shift your eating habits to adhere more closely to the Paleotech Diet. This will take you a long way in helping you reach and maintain your "normal" weight. In order for you to follow the Paleotech Diet, however, you have to give up some of your toxic dietary practices. You must understand that eating certain foods is inconsistent with achieving the fat-burning goals of the High-Tech Body. For instance, something as simple as one soda a day can be extremely harmful. A study published in the British medical journal *The Lancet* (February 17, 2001) showed that children who drink sugary sodas are at high risk of becoming obese, and that for every additional serving of soft drink consumed, the risk of becoming obese increases by about 50 percent.

Habits like eating foods—especially nufoods—in front of the television also contribute to weight gain and obesity. Nufoods, as I covered in the chapter on the Paleotech Diet, disrupt the body's ability to burn fat effectively. We now know that the overconsumption of fat itself seems to increase triglycerides in the blood, apparently activating receptor centers deep within the brain that open appetite. So, eating fat itself, especially the highly concentrated fat in nufoods, seems to tell the body that what it should do is continue to eat even more, destroying your ability to regulate your own appetite.

When you eliminate nufoods from your diet and substitute healthy Paleotech foods, you automatically help control your insulin, glucagon, and cortisol levels.

A QUICK NOTE ABOUT FAT

There are basically two types of fat in our bodies:

- **White fat:** is the insulating fat layer under our skin that stores excess calories as fat. This is the stuff we want to get rid of.

- **Brown fat:** is a special type of fat tissue that burns excess calories. Brown fat keeps the body warm by releasing the energy stored in fat as heat. It is believed that the setpoint is controlled by this tissue. Hibernating animals and human infants have relatively large amounts of brown fat. Unfortunately, brown fat decreases with age, which may account for the fact that it's more difficult to lose weight as you get older.

  However, the December 2000 issue of *New Scientist* magazine reported that researchers have found a way to turn white-fat cells in rats into brown-fat cells. Of course, they're still working on achieving the same effect in humans.

Steps 4 to 5: Paleofitness

Once again, we have to return to our Paleolithic ancestors in order to understand the importance of exercise in fat burning. Studies have shown over and over again that exercise is an important component of controlling hormones, especially insulin. Our ancestors didn't know this, nor did they have to worry about it, because exercise was a natural part of their existence; their survival, in fact, depended on it. They needed to be able to walk long distances in the face of changing climates and food availability; they had to run to hunt for food; they had to be strong to carry game back to others in their tribes and to do all the other tasks associated with their strenuous daily lives.

In other words, they were forced to be fit.

We don't have those same outside influences. We have to force ourselves to be fit. We have to exercise for the express purposes of balancing hormones, and thereby managing body weight and fat. Without exercise, the discussion on controlling weight stops.

Trying to lose weight permanently through food manipulation alone has been shown over and over to be an antiquated approach and is simply a bust all by itself; you'll have to become fit and train to achieve fat loss. Everything, every book, journal, and article you read today, *any study* that has anything useful to say about weight loss will emphasize just this point. The most successful means of controlling weight and fat is a combination of prudent eating and fitness.

At the University of Wisconsin, a review of research in the field found that thirty minutes or more of low-intensity exercise could burn more calories and body fat than brief high-intensity exercise that's sustained for only minutes. Further, studies show that calorie burning continues after you stop exercising, perhaps for even longer than was previously thought. Dr. Ronald Barr at the National Institute of Health at Oslo studied the effects of exercise intensity and duration. He found that exercising for thirty minutes causes the metabolic rate to increase by an extra 150 calories more than normal over a twelve-hour period. That means you're burning calories both during and after your workout. Dr. Barr also found that the body increases its use of fat after exercise by 300 percent. It seems the harder your workout intensity, the greater the postexercise fat burning.

Aerobic exercise turns out to be critical in the management of the hunger mechanism, the storage of fat in cells, and keeping you in the lower range of your setpoint, controlling insulin levels in blood, and helping your body accurately adjust caloric intake to output. In a *New York Times* article titled "One-Two Punch for Losing Pounds: Exercise and Careful Diet" (October 17, 2000), Dr. Peter Wood, professor emeritus of medicine at Stanford University, said, "We evolved as an active species and our 'appestats' by which we adjust food intake with body needs, seem to function best when we are active."

Exercise changes the way the body processes food, making it easier for it to be used for energy than to be stored as fat. When you're active, the fat in a meal tends to be burned for energy. When you're sedentary, the amount of fat that's burned goes way down and winds up being stored (in all the wrong places) instead of being used by the muscles.

Preferred forms of aerobic activity are:

- walking

- running

- spinning

- cycling

- hiking

- aerobic classes

- skiing

EXERCISE AND ALL-AROUND HEALTH A key point here is that exercise has proven to be an important preventative factor in many diseases, from heart disease to diabetes to cancer. This relates directly to how effective exercise is in slowing aging and maintaining functionality. *Exercise is a whole body phenomenon*, meaning it does more than just make your muscles stronger, it slows down the aging of your body. It affects everything: your cardiovascular system, your immune system, your musculoskeletal system, and your emotional stability. Even your very cells are affected.

Everyone wishes there were a magic pill that would allow you to look fantastic without exercising. "That would be great from a vanity point of view," says fitness expert Jonny Bowden. "But it would not be great from a health point of view. Even if weight is out of the picture, there are still measurable, demonstrable, life-enhancing, age-retarding effects to exercise. It still benefits your immune system and cardiovascular system. It still increases your serotonin levels. It still extends your life.

"When it comes right down to it, would you really want such a pill? What if I told you that I could invent a pill so that you could have a good relationship without sex? Sure, you could save some time . . . but it's not all about time. In the same way, it's not all about weight."

Exercise is aerobic if it makes the heart and lungs work harder to meet the muscles' need for oxygen. Aerobic exercise uses the lower part of your body, thighs, and buttocks because the bigger the muscle, the greater the volume of calories burned.

How much exercise is appropriate? According to Covert Bailey, one of the world's great authorities on weight control and fitness, the answer is: often—seven days a week if possible. He recommends that, if lifestyle permits, you exercise two or three times a day for fifteen or twenty minutes at a time. Other experts suggest thirty to forty-five minutes of moderately intense activity (like vigorous walking) every day.

When exercising aerobically, try to work up to a heart rate between 130 and 150 beats a minute, depending on your age (if you're young, go for the higher heart rate; as you age, your goal is the lower number). This is your target heart rate (THR). Reaching it, and keeping it there for thirty to forty-five minutes, will put you into your fat-burning mode.

In addition, it appears that adding muscle through weight training is a second and necessary tool for weight control. Weight training is an example of anaerobic exercise, which does not need extra oxygen. This type of exercise uses up the food stored in the muscles quickly, often within three or four minutes. Many people (especially women) are afraid to pursue weight training because they think it will make them heavier, in terms of pounds. However, as Cliff Sheats says in his book *Lean Bodies*, "Weight training develops lean body mass (muscle), and the more lean mass you have, the faster your metabolism." For those trying to drop weight and looking to maintain their lean muscle mass as they get older (which means all of us), weight training is essential because:

- Muscle tissue is seventy times more metabolically active than fat.

- Muscle uses far more calories than the same amount of fat tissue.

- Muscle is the most energy-active tissue in the body.

- For every pound of muscle you have, the better you burn fat. For every pound of new muscle you put on, you'll burn fifty to one hundred more calories per day.

It's difficult to make universal recommendations for starting a muscle-building, strengthening, or toning program. If at all possible, seek out professional advice and coaching. Get a trainer, do it right. You don't have to hire a personal trainer to be your partner at every workout. Find someone who will work with you two or three times to help you determine the best workout for your goals and current fitness level. This will minimize injuries and maximize your gains.

It's important to point out that any results you are looking for must always consider the "complex group of dynamics" referred to earlier in this chapter. Weight loss is different for men than for women. It becomes more difficult as you age, for a variety of reasons that I'll call the *inertia of aging*. You naturally lose about one half pound of muscle each year after the age of twenty-five (if you don't stay fit). That's about five or six pounds each decade, so that by age fifty-six you've lost 25 to 30 percent of your muscle mass and strength. And you know what will fill up all that space—FAT!

Step 6: Sleep and Stress Control

Here's information you've probably never heard before: *the amount of sleep you get has a direct correlation to weight gain and obesity.* Numerous studies have linked a failure to receive adequate sleep, especially a part of the sleep cycle called rapid eye movement (REM) sleep, with weight gain. In an apparently vicious cycle, sleep problems can contribute to weight gain and obesity—and weight gain and obesity can interfere with sleep. Dr. Jennifer Peszka, and her colleagues at the University of Southern Mississippi in Hattiesburg, studied 163 patients as part of a sleep-disorder study. They found that patients who got the least REM sleep, the deepest part of the sleep cycle, were the heaviest. They found, conversely, that patients who got more REM sleep after treatment lost weight, and that those who showed the biggest increase in REM sleep lost the most weight.

I have seen the truth of this in my own practice. A client in her mid-twenties came to me, concerned about her weight. She seemed to be doing everything right. She was eating properly. She was on an intensive exercise program: she met with a trainer five days a week and exercised on her own the other two days. In fact, she was getting up at 5:30 A.M. to exercise so she could be at the office by 7:30. She would work all day, and then, three nights a week, attend college classes, come home, and do her homework. Needless to say, she was getting only about four hours of sleep a night.

She thought she was doing everything possible to control her weight, but in reality she was cheating on sleep. It became increasingly clear that unless she made changes to her lifestyle, she would suffer the consequences found in the University of Southern Mississippi study.

You should not undervalue sleep as a component of the Healthy High-Tech Body. If you are underrested, overly tired during the day, wake up at night, and (here's the important part) told that you snore—get help! Check out the possibility that you may have sleep apnea. According to Dr. William C. Dement, author of *The Promise of Sleep*, nearly 40 percent of the population has sleep apnea, a condition where you actually stop breathing several times during the night. It is often coupled with severe snoring. Dr. Peszka's findings suggest, as do numerous others', that apnea contributes to weight gain, at least in part by disrupting REM sleep.

And here's another problem: by the time men reach the age of forty-five, they have nearly lost the ability to fall into deep sleep, according to Eve Van Cauter, professor of medicine at the University of Chicago, who led a study on sleep, published in the *Journal of the American Medical Association* (August 16, 2000). The study also correlated this change in sleep with a drop in human growth hormone of nearly 75 percent. Human growth hormone (hGH) is produced by the pituitary gland and is important to the growth process from birth through adolescence. We already know that a deficiency of hGH impacts on, well . . . everything, especially by increasing the volume of fat and abdominal obesity we store, and by reducing muscle mass and strength. A drop in your natural production of hGH is a direct pathway to producing flab.

According to Dr. Van Cauter, you can increase hGH by increasing "deep sleep." Researchers, however, have yet to determine "the chicken or the egg" in this conundrum: does the quality of sleep influence the production of hormones, or are the changes in hormones responsible for the changes in sleep? As in most chicken-and-egg conundrums, it really doesn't matter. What matters is that you realize the incredible benefits of adequate sleep, an essential goal for achieving a Healthy High-Tech Body.

Another essential goal is controlling stress. Here's another chicken-and-egg conundrum: stress influences the food you eat, and the food you eat influences stress. You might experience an increase in appetite when you're stressed out. If so, you may be suffering from hyperglycemia, or high blood sugar. Your cortisol levels may be high. Essentially, the body is accessing and burning the fuel available, in the food you're eating, rather than properly accessing stored fat. When that happens, you try to keep yourself energized by eating sugar and carbs.

On the other hand, stress may cause you to eat less often, but with larger meals. That might be a sign that stress is making your thyroid and adrenal glands sluggish, and slowing down your metabolic activity. So you may also look to sugar and even caffeine to keep yourself going.

Whatever your reaction, the stress itself and stress-based eating cause disturbances in a hormone called cholecystokinin (CCK), the substance that signals the brain to make you feel full. When you're under stress, you tend to eat faster; therefore, you don't give CCK enough time to send its signals to the brain. Your stoplight system is out of order, and you'll eat more than you should.

Step 7: Nutraceuticals for Burning Fat

The main thing supplements help accomplish is providing chemical support for regulating appetite and for burning accumulated fat. There are many "fat burners" on the market. They work in a variety of ways with varying degrees of effectiveness. The term we'll use here to describe "fat burning" is *thermogenesis*. Thermogenesis is the creation of heat from the stored energy that is fat.

The primary ingredient in the most successful products on the market that produce thermogenesis is mahuang/ephedra, an herb with a five-thousand-year history of successful use. There has been much controversy about ephedra's benefits and safety as a dietary supplement. Most recently, key testimony at a conference sponsored by the Department of Health and Human Services Office of Women's Health provided overwhelming, let me repeat *overwhelming*, evidence by consumers, treating physicians, scientists, organizations, research consulting firms (Cantox Health Science International), and trial studies (both at Columbia and Harvard universities), showing that the use of up to 90 milligrams of ephedra a day is safe and effective as a tool for weight management. (As always, consult with your physician before using products containing ephedra.)

The secondary ingredient (for the purposes of fat burning) is caffeine, usually extracted from the guarana nut.

The third ingredient important for fat burning is usually white willow bark/salicin extract.

These three compounds constitute the base ingredients of the most successful fat burners on the market. They constitute a "stack" that, added together, produce a fat-burning synergy whose safety and effectiveness have been highly documented.

CAFFEINE? In chapter 2, caffeine was to be eliminated from your diet. So how can we advocate its use here as a fat-burning ingredient? Because in this context you're going to use caffeine temporarily, in small amounts, for its targeted effect of making ephedra work more effectively. Some supplements actually use green tea extract in place of caffeine. It's the synergy of supplements' ingredients that make them effective for burning fat.

Here are some of the most effective over-the-counter fat-burning products:

- **Xenadrine** by Cytodine Technologies

- **Thermicore CRT** by MET-Rx

- **Triphetamine** by Pharmologics

- **Ripped Fuel** by Twinlabs (with or without mahuang)

My second line of attack-fat products for additional support:

- CLA fatty acid products (**CLA FUEL** by Twinlabs)

- St. John's wort extract (**Hyperimed** by Phytopharmica)

- **Energenics** by Metagenics

- **NADH** by Enada

My third line of support products:

- Meal bars, such as **Protein Revolution Bars, Pure Protein, MET-Rx** bars (great for between-meal snacks)

- Whey-based shake powders, such as **Designer Protein, Isopure, Myoplex, MET-Rx, Labrada Lean Body, FuelPlex** by Twinlabs

IMPORTANT NOTE The above products should be used only after consultation with your doctor. There are risks involved in using any supplementation that affects metabolism, especially if you are taking prescription drugs or over-the-counter medications. It is extremely important to consult your doctor if you have any medical condition such as high blood pressure or diabetes.

If you think that sitting back and taking supplements is going to do it for you . . . *forget it!* These supplements should be used as part of a supervised weight management program. However, these are the products that I've determined are the most effective for the purposes of weight loss.

There are diet drugs that work (available only by prescription and medical supervision required).

If you have severe weight problems and have experienced no results from all the other components listed in this chapter, talk to your doctor about the possibility of using prescription drugs. Although this should not be your first line of defense, here are some of the available drugs your doctor may recommend:

- **Sibutramine**, also known as Meridia. This drug works on the brain, specifically on two different neurotransmitter pathways, reducing food intake and increasing energy expenditure. It can be used for up to a year.

- **Diethylpropion**, also known as Tenuate, is considered medically quite safe for up to twenty-four weeks to produce weight loss.

- **Mazindol**, also known as Sanorex, is an effective appetite suppressant.

- **Phentermine**, also known as Fastin and Ionamin, is used as an appetite suppressant.

IMPORTANT NOTE These are powerful drugs that may have side effects. Used under proper medical supervision they can be of great help in controlling appetite and losing weight. Which drug(s) you take should be determined after checking with your doctor. It's also important to ask your doctor to test you for thyroid problems, in which case you may need different medications. There are other hormone deficiencies, such as DHEA or testosterone, that can also contribute to weight gain and difficulty in losing weight. Your doctor can test for these deficiencies as well, and determine if you need medication to correct the problem.

In my work I've come across several brilliant doctors, working with medications in different combinations for successful appetite and weight control, often in the most stubborn of situations. In New York City, for example, Dr. Ron Ruden, author of *The Craving Brain,* treats weight problems and eating disorders caused by imbalances of brain chemicals. He uses a pharmacological model to deal with patients; that is, he often treats depression (by prescribing antidepressants) at the same time he is dealing with issues of weight loss. Hormone imbalances are often accompanied by emotional and behavioral issues that also need to be addressed. It may be necessary to seek help in those areas as well (a good place to start for behavioral and emotional support is *Shape Up!* by Jonny Bowden).

Ann Louise Gittleman's Fat Flush

There are times when you may decide you want to rev up your metabolism and jumpstart your fat-burning program. You can do that by using the "Two-Week Fat Flush" featured in Ann Louise Gittleman's book *The Fat Flush Plan* (McGraw-Hill, 2002). Gittleman is an authority on human health and nutrition and a prolific author. For the purposes of the High-Tech Body, I've made some dietary modifications and supplement recommendations that are closer to my view of what to use during a fat-loss program. You can find more information in Gittleman's book and by visiting www.iVillage.com on the Internet. There you'll find a library of information, message boards, and additional support information on the classic Fat Flush.

The purpose of the fourteen-day Fat-Flush diet is twofold. First, it is a very good cleansing and detoxifying break for your system, making it easier for your metabolism to burn fat. Second, it will jump-start your weight loss by reducing accumulated toxins, bloating, and fluid retention. It is a great basic form of detoxification that reduces congestion in your liver from chemicals, drugs, bacteria, and any other toxins that might be residing there.

Diet

The foods you'll eat for breakfast, lunch, and dinner are from the following groups only: lean protein, vegetables, oils, fruits, cleansing cocktails (see below).

Lean protein: Choose from lean animal, seafood, and vegetarian sources like fish, turkey, and eggs. Protein helps to stabilize blood sugar.

Vegetables: Unlimited low-glycemic vegetables, cooked or raw. Remember to choose from a rainbow of colors—the more colorful the better. Veggies are cleansing as well as rich in antioxidants, vitamins, and natural enzymes. Many are a good source of fiber too.

Fruits: Limited portions. Choose from an array of colorful, low-glycemic fruits like berries or grapefruit. Fruits contain enzymes to help cleanse your system.

Fats and oils: Special fat-burning oils and supplements, which contain the essential fatty acids. Flax oil is the primary choice.

Cleansing cocktail: An elixir, which acts as a diuretic and cleanser for bodily systems. It also contains powerful enzymes to help block fat absorption. The drink is made from a soluble fiber (like psyllium) blend to help augment fat excretion. Twice a day it is mixed with purified water and unsweetened cranberry juice.

Some Suggestions

- Avoid most seasonings and extra salt that's added to foods, simply to avoid water retention and to speed up elimination.

- Drink 8 ounces of water, 6 to 8 times a day. Water is the eternal cleanser. It is a superb body hydrator and keeps the brain alert.

- You may eat allowable sources of protein whenever you want throughout the day, as well as designated portions of fruit and unlimited vegetables from those listed in Gittleman's book *The Fat Flush Plan*. You can make vegetable soups and salads; you can grill, broil, bake, or steam your vegetables—be as creative as you want. It's architecturally clean and simple. You have plenty of leeway and it works beautifully. I know because I've used it many times myself and have recommended it to countless clients.

My Customized Sample Menu

Upon arising

Cleansing cocktail

Breakfast

2- to 3-egg omelet with vegetables (such as steamed or stir-fried spinach). Add olive oil. If hungry, add a small cup of fruit

Midmorning snack

Fruit

Before lunch

3 ounces water (10 to 20 minutes before the meal)

Lunch

Broiled swordfish or broiled tuna steak

Large mixed green salad, olive oil, squeezed lemon, sprinkled with a little balsamic vinegar

8 ounces water

Midafternoon

8 ounces water, cleansing cocktail or fruit

Dinner

Chicken, baked, broiled, or grilled

Assortment of cooked vegetables, such as asparagus—4 ounces

Small salad with olive oil and balsamic vinegar

Midevening

Fruit or long-life cocktail

Using This Menu

You can use the preceding example as a basic menu guide. Substitute foods from the different food groups for daily variety. Adjust fluid intake to suit your schedule.

Nutraceuticals

You can enhance the effects of the Fat Flush by incorporating a fat-burning supplement or two along with a good-quality source of omega-6 fatty acids to help reduce inflammation while you are on the Fat Flush. More on these in the next chapter, along with my list of recommended fat-management products.

You can use the Fat Flush for one to two weeks. It will clean out your system and get your weight loss started. Repeat every three or four months. After the flush, add the other foods within the Paleotech Diet guidelines.

Final Note

Achieving a Healthy High-Tech Body is an ongoing goal. We are in a constant battle between our evolution and our civilization. We are built to burn fat under very different circumstances than those in which we now find ourselves. Losing weight is, unfortunately, not easy.

As you've probably realized by now, there is no one secret to fat burning. It's a package deal. It's not just food, not just exercise, not just sleep, not just supplements and medication. It's the synergy of all these factors that will lead to your personal Healthy High-Tech Body.

The Paleo Package

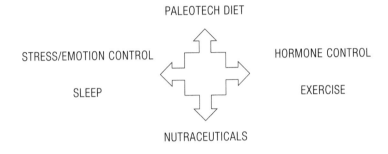

PALEOTECH DIET

STRESS/EMOTION CONTROL   HORMONE CONTROL

SLEEP   EXERCISE

NUTRACEUTICALS

5 High-Tech Nutraceuticals

The A list

Why do you need supplements (or **nutraceuticals**, as I prefer to call them)? If you follow the Paleotech Diet guidelines, if you exercise, get enough sleep, and keep stress under control, shouldn't that be enough to keep your body regulated? Can't you reach High-Tech health "naturally"?

Not if we're talking about enhancing and improving efficiency. It's like going from New York to California. I know I can get there "naturally," using only my own two feet. But if I want to maximize efficiency, I'm going to take advantage of the technology of aerodynamics, and I'm going to fly there. There are limits imposed on me by life and work, not to mention my aging body, that impede my own ability to walk those thousands of miles.

In terms of health, there are limits imposed on us all by age, genetics, and circumstances. These limits are not the same as they once were. Used to be, we'd live to a ripe old age of fifty, fifty-five, maybe sixty. Now we're living to seventy, eighty, ninety, one hundred. That's a much longer amount of time for cells to divide and replicate, providing many more chances for things to go wrong. We want to reduce the chances for mistakes and mishaps. It's like owning a much-loved car. As it gets older, and the machinery runs down, the more you're going to have to "fuss" with it to keep it in great running shape. To keep our bodies in great running shape, we use supplements.

The closer we get to maximum life expectancy, the greater the push against the battle of the aging body. Supplements are part of the advancing technology allowing us to win that battle.

In a way, this chapter is preaching to the choir. Most of us already use some kind of supplementation; in fact, more than 60 percent of Americans regularly consume a dietary supplement. Media reports, articles, books, journals, news segments, and Internet sites continually promote the use of supplements in a wide range of applications. As a result, most of us have read or heard that the consumption of the right supplements in proper potencies can reduce the risks of contracting cancer, cataracts, cardiovascular problems, Alzheimer's, and numerous other diseases associated with aging.

There is also a large and quickly expanding field of supplementation that is used for physical enhancement, rather than disease prevention. These supplements increase muscle mass, improve agility, and help maintain mental function.

There are hundreds, if not thousands, of supplements available to you today. There are complete books on the subject. This chapter doesn't try to cover all of them, or talk about many of the ones we already know about (and many of us already take) like vitamin C, vitamin E, and simple antioxidants.

Here, we're talking about supplements designed to *raise efficiency,* to keep the body working in top form. The products listed here are on the cutting edge. They're safe, effective Healthy High-Tech Body solutions.

Most vitamins and supplements do not cause any health problems themselves. However, excessive use of individual products can be unhealthy; you should always check with your healthcare provider or nutritionist before taking any new supplement, especially if you are taking prescription or over-the-counter medications.

Much of the rationale for taking supplementation in the context of the Healthy High-Tech Body is to generate and maintain "youthful health." There are research foundations, organizations, clinical studies, government studies, university studies, and independent researchers from a multitude of disciplines (medical and otherwise) involved in measuring the impact that supplement use can make on quality of life and upgrading your body's health. This development of the field of supplements and nutraceuticals owes a great deal to health pioneer Dr. Steven Levine, founder of Nutricology and one of the first to research and make public the effects of free radicals on health and the role of antioxidants in containing their damage. Another pioneer is Saul Kent, executive director of the Life Extension Foundation, an organization dedicated to the "investigation of scientific methods of preventing and treating disease, aging, and death." The foundation also funds pioneering scientific research aimed at achieving an indefinitely extended healthy human life span.

From the foundation comes the following list of causes of the diseases of aging *that are controllable.* Here are nine of the most common:

1. Chronic inflammation: both outward and inward, from arthritis to damage in brain cells and arterial walls. As time goes on, inflammation is being linked to more and more problems; everything from heart valve failure to senility has been linked to the chronic inflammatory cascade so often seen in aging humans.

2. Glycosylation: this is where sugar/glucose molecules and protein molecules bind in the body to form nonfunctioning structures (remember AGEs?). Glycosylation is most evident in senile dementia, stiffening of the arterial system, and degenerative diseases of the eye.

3. Hormone imbalance: aging creates a severe hormone imbalance that is a contributing cause to many diseases associated with aging, including depression, osteoporosis, coronary artery disease, and loss of libido.

4. Fatty acid imbalance: the effects of fatty acid imbalances may manifest as irregular heartbeat, joint degeneration, dry skin, hypercoagulation, and a host of other ailments. This occurs with alteration in enzyme pathways that cannot convert essential fatty acids into the specific nutrients the body needs to perform.

5. DNA mutations: both synthetic and natural compounds mutate cellular DNA and cause cancer cells to form. Aging cells lose their DNA gene repair mechanisms; the result is that DNA genetic damage can cause cells to proliferate out of control, often forming cancerous tumors.

6. Immune dysfunction: our aging and stressed immune systems lose their ability to attack bacteria, viruses, and cancer cells. In aging humans, excessive levels of dangerous cytokines (proteins that regulate immunity and inflammation) are produced that cause the immune system to turn on its host and create autoimmune diseases, such as lupus, diabetes, and rheumatoid arthritis.

7. Excitotoxicity: the aging brain loses control over its release of neurotransmitters, such as glutamate and dopamine; this results in devastating brain cell damage and destruction.

8. Circulatory deficit: microcapillary circulation to the brain, eyes, and skin is impaired as part of normal aging. The result is that disorders of the eye (macular degeneration, cataracts, glaucoma) are the number-one age-related degenerative diseases. Major and ministrokes are other common problems associated with circulatory deficits to the brain.

9. Oxidative stress: free radicals are unstable molecules that have been implicated in most diseases associated with aging. Antioxidants are the supplements used to protect against free radical–induced cell damage.

The complete list of controllable causes of aging, plus further support documentation and data, is available through the Life Extension Foundation, their website (www.oz.lef.org), and their *Directory of Life Extension Technologies.* I would also direct you to the foundation's medical reference, *Disease, Prevention and Treatment,* for the most comprehensive and encyclopedic review of innovative supplemental, drug, and medical treatments.

Now, remember that I'm talking about "controllability." You may not be able to prevent every possible disease of aging. But because of the ever-expanding field of nutraceuticals, you can control many of them.

There are many single supplements available to "control" varying aspects of health. There are also combinations of supplements, vitamins, minerals, amino acids, herbs, and chemicals that when mixed together produce a richer, deeper effect in the desired category.

What are the categories of supplements that are important to the Healthy High-Tech Body? Although the following list isn't exhaustive, it is highly targeted and focused. It can be difficult to separate nutraceuticals into categories, because they often have more than one function; they very often operate along multiple trajectories, crosscutting back and forth. For example, SAMe (an amino acid) is used primarily as an antidepressant (although "mood brightener" is probably a better term); however, it also helps prevent and reverse liver disease and may be effective in the treatment of chronic pain. As a result, some products will show up in multiple categories. Others will show up numerous times throughout the book in pertinent sections.

Unless otherwise noted, follow the manufacturers' recommended dosages when using these products, or follow the recommendations of your healthcare practitioner.

Not every nutraceutical listed here will be appropriate for you. If you're in your twenties or thirties, you may need fewer of them. As you get older, the benefits of nutraceuticals increase. So you need to read through the various sections, find products that apply to your individual situation, discuss them with your healthcare provider, and then design your appropriate Healthy High-Tech Body program.

Basics

LIFE EXTENSION MIX TABLETS, CAPSULES, AND POWDERS BY LIFE EXTENSION

This product is the "Swiss Army knife" of nutraceuticals, containing eighty-nine super-high potency ingredients that target each of the *causes* of the diseases of aging listed above and more. Its broad spectrum and shotgun mechanism target every-thing from inhibiting glycosylation to improving microcapillary circulation. What's in it? The kitchen sink: a wide range of longevity nutrients; phytochemicals, such as lycopene; herbs; vegetable extracts; primary and secondary antioxidants; vitamins; and more.

PERM A VITE POWDER BY NUTRICOLOGY

There are many great bowel nourishment products on the market; this one is a key product for cleaning out and normalizing lower bowel function. It is a state-of-the-art repair product. You need a properly functioning colon under all conditions to have a highly functional life. The reasons are obvious. The intestinal lining becomes damaged through years of bad eating habits like consuming too many nufoods. Add in the use and abuse of medications (like antibiotics) and alcohol, and you end up killing off all your important intestinal flora. A healthy human colon contains lots of bacteria (most of them are good for you), performing all sorts of important functions to keep you healthy and alive. Perm A vite promotes gastric healing; improves the gastrointestinal environment in which healthy bacteria can thrive; enhances the detoxification of the colon; and pro-vides nutrition for the *villi* (tiny projections that

> **LYCOPENE** Lycopene is a phytochemical found in tomatoes that makes them red. Lycopene offers protection against cancer and may be ten times stronger than beta-carotene. It also protects arteries and the heart against plaque formation. The most protective effect comes from a very high consumption of tomatoes, best if cooked or juiced. Due to the fact that we simply don't consume cooked tomatoes in high enough amounts, taking lycopene in supplement form is a Healthy High-Tech Body must!

cover the lining) of the colon, "sweeping" the gastrointestinal tract. This product is essential in returning your colon to good health. It comes as a powder that you can add to water, juice, or shakes. It is a top-flight source of fiber. You can strengthen its effects by matching it up with any number of high-end "friendly bacteria" powders to replenish the intestinal flora.

Note: These beneficial bacteria are an invaluable component in the prevention of many illnesses and unhealthy conditions. If you do not support them as part of achieving a long, healthy functional life, you're missing an indispensable component in achieving this goal.

NATREN INTESTINAL BACTERIA BY NATREN
SYMBIOTICS BY NUTRICOLOGY

Both these companies make products that I use in my practice and recommend for intestinal health.

Natren makes three different strains of helpful bacteria (superacidophilus, bifido, and bulgaricum), which are available individually and that I recommend be used in rotation (replenish the flora in your colon using one strain until you complete its contents, then rotate on to the next, and so on). Natren also makes a strain of bacteria specifically for children, which is especially effective for kids who suffer from recurring ear infections and like problems. It is highly recommended for children who were not breast fed.

Symbiotics is one product that contains nine strains of probiotics, plus additional ingredients that enable these probiotics to do a better job in your colon. This is a vital product for the Healthy High-Tech Body; I consider it an essential basic.

PROGREENS BY NUTRICOLOGY

This is available in both powder form and capsule.

Progreens by Nutricology is a superfood, combining a broad base of nutritional grasses, sea vegetables, algae, fibers, herbs, and additional probiotics. It is an elegantly designed food product providing many nutrients that are simply overlooked or have been dropped from our diet as a result of our overdemanding lives. It is a great base to start your day with when mixed with water or juice.

SHAKING IT UP Over the years I have become fond of designing shakes for me and my clients. Shakes make it easy to combine any number of nutrients in one "thick" drink and to use it as a meal replacement, usually breakfast. The bad news is that you may have to doctor the shake to make it palatable; oftentimes you'll wind up trading taste for convenience. You get everything you need in one shot, but you gotta hold your nose.

Protein Powders

DESIGNER PROTEIN BY THE NEXT CORP.
FUELPLEX BY TWINLABS
MET-Rx BY MET-Rx
MYOPLEX BY EAS

Protein powders come in many variations. Some are egg based, some are soy based, and some (my favorites) are whey based. Shakes are a great way to start off most mornings. Quality whey-based powders, besides providing the macronutrients for building muscle and body tissues, also deliver a vast array of immune support nutrients, such as naturally occurring immunoglobulins. They are also rich in antioxidants, especially those involved in liver detoxification. The whey powders that I recommend are also high in protein value and low in carbohydrates and fats. The whey shake powders listed above are continually being tweaked and improved. Designer Protein, for example, has added ZMA to its formula, a novel combination of zinc monomethionine and magnesium aspartate that increases both muscle and power, apparently by affecting growth hormone levels.

These shakes are highly functional foods that can be used as part of weight loss or muscle-building programs, as well as part of your general maintenance program.

DHA FATTY ACID BY THORNE RESEARCH, LEF FOUNDATION, NUTRICOLOGY, TWINLABS

Docosahexaenoic acid (DHA) is an omega-3 fatty acid. Omegas are a special class of polyunsaturated fats, some of which, like DHA, are considered very valuable for human health. The body makes DHA from the essential fatty acid linoleic acid, but the main dietary sources are fish and fish oils. Since most people don't get enough fish oil in their diets, DHA can be an excellent supplemental source (at least one gram per day). DHA is a multitasking product with measurable effects on everything from arthritis to blood clotting, depression, and systemic inflammation. According to *The Directory of Life Extension Technologies 2000*, it may even slow down aspects of normal aging through mechanisms similar to calorie restriction.

Energy and Brain Performance, Smart Nutrients and Mood

There are a number of excellent products on the market that perform many functions, affecting both mental and physical efficiency. Some nutrients that elevate energy simply cross over categorically, affecting brain performance while elevating mood; improving athletic performance and sexual endurance, and so on, traveling all over the "performance" map. The boundaries may blur between what may be good for "energy," however you define it, and what may be good for your brain.

I'm suggesting that if you can improve everything all at the same time, the coactive effect produces a heightened state of energy. (Note that energy does not necessarily equal power; power is a more distinct effect that I will address later on.) There are several hormonal systems that are central to the production of energy; for instance, your adrenal glands and your thyroid. The products in this category will help these glands, and others responsible for generating energy, to increase their efficiency—which is the goal of using these supplements.

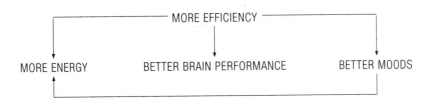

CHOLINE COCKTAIL BY TWINLABS

The human brain has a voracious appetite for choline (more on this in chapter 7, "The Power Brain"). Choline is a B vitamin, classified as an essential nutrient for humans. It plays multiple roles in brain efficiency and function and a crucial role in cognitive development before and after birth. As we get older, choline becomes an important component in the synthesis of the neurotransmitter acetylcholine, which is vital for thought, memory, and sleep, and is involved in the control of movements. The production of acetylcholine declines with age and is abnormally low in people who have Alzheimer's disease.

Choline Cocktail contains an important ingredient called phosphatidylserine, yet another essential brain nutrient with broad applications from mood to memory boosting; it also appears to reduce anxiety and help protect the body from the more damaging aspects of stress. There are additional ingredients in Choline Cocktail, such as huperzine, which is an herb known to protect against Alzheimer's, and DMAE, a brain-stimulatory vitaminlike compound. Choline Cocktail comes in an orange-flavored powder, which can be added to your morning shake. You can also mix it in juice and drink a glass along with your breakfast. Choline Cocktail also contains ginkgo biloba. It appears that ginkgo is not as effective by itself as when it's combined with other nutrients, such as the ones in the Choline Cocktail.

BRAIN WAVE PLUS BY NUTRICOLOGY

This product is supremely elegant in its construction. Below are some of its ingredients, involved in supporting a variety of mental functions and underlying neurocognitive performance, such as clarity of mind and memory:

- acetyl-L-carnitine: ALC is an amino acid that maintains the cell's energy. It has been shown to protect the brain against age-related degeneration and to improve memory, cognition, and mood. This is an effective product to use even by itself (however, don't take this product if you have epilepsy; you're already too sensitive to neural stimulation). Acetyl-L-carnitine also protects against the buildup of lipofuscion in the brain, a fatty acid that deposits in the nerve cells and is associated with a reduction of cognitive powers.

- vinpocetine: a powerful memory enhancer that has been used in Europe for many years. It facilitates cerebral metabolism by improving microcirculation (blood flow), stepping up brain-cell ATP production (the energy molecule), and increasing the utilization of glucose and oxygen. This is a potent cognitive enhancer that is used by doctors to treat acute stroke, inner ear problems, and even headaches. This product can also be taken separately from Brain Wave Plus.

- CDP Choline: a very special type of choline that readily penetrates the blood-brain barrier. It activates the synthesis of critical components in cell membranes, boosts levels of neurotransmitters such as acetylcholine, and enhances brain energy metabolism.

- DMAE: a memory-enhancing substance. It is also a safe and effective brain stimulant. Cellular degradation has been proposed as a primary mechanism of aging, and DMAE is common to a number of compounds known to stabilize cellular membranes. In Europe it is combined with the drug Centrophenoxine (more on this in the Power Brain chapter) to boost cognitive function.

- huperzine A: mental improvement associated with this herb stems from the compound's ability to inhibit the breakdown of acetylcholine, a brain chemical essential to memory. This compound appears to have the power to sharpen the mind and potentially ward off the devastating effects of Alzheimer's, particularly at its early stages.

NADH BY THE ENADA CORP.

Reduced B-nicotinamide adenine dinucleotide (NADH) is an extraordinarily complex compound with multiple applications. It is a coenzyme, which means it is a substance that makes it possible for certain enzymes to do their work in the body. It is one of most powerful products on the market today with the most uniform impact on energy—lifting both your mood and your spirit. Rather than producing the hollow lift of stimulants such as caffeine, this product actually increases and improves energenic performance in both your body and your brain. NADH has been clinically tested for a wide range of neuropsychiatric and brain disorders, with remarkable results. It is currently being researched for its positive effects on Alzheimer's, Parkinson's, chronic fatigue syndrome, and clinical depression. It is extremely effective for improving athletic performance, memory, and cognitive function; it functions as an antioxidant and enhances the cellular immune system.

There are many, many reasons any one individual may be lacking energy. Yet because NADH is so involved in the production of energy neurotransmitters and enzymes, it can "correct" a variety of flaws. There is also a new version of NADH that is great for mitigating jet lag, called Enada Alert. This is a terrific product if you want to stay on top of your game.

PROENDORPHIN BY PHARMALOGIC

Proendorphin is extremely effective at increasing energy and endurance. I would also qualify it as a mood brightener. It comes in an effervescent "fizzy powder" delivery system. It is a novel configuration of vitamins, amino acids, and herbs that, in combination, are especially useful before workouts and around that 3:00 or 4:00 afternoon slump. Instead of trying to get a lift from sugar or unhealthy carbohydrates, Proendorphin does a much better job. (And, as a side note, it's very good for hangovers!)

ENERGENICS BY THE METAGENICS CORP

This is an extremely well-designed product for improving your *resting metabolic rate*, or the rate at which you burn calories at rest. This product is especially effective if you have low thyroid function (which can be determined by medical analysis). It's also great for helping an aging metabolism perform better.

VINCACLEAR BY LIFE ENHANCEMENT

This is vinpocetine in combination with several other nutrients that facilitate its uptake by the brain.

MEMORACTIVE BY THORNE RESEARCH

A powerful brain formulation that includes bacopa monniera extract. Bacopa monniera is a plant from India which, in extract form (bacosides), plays a protective role in the synaptic functions of the nerves in the hippocampus. Clinical studies confirm that bacosides can revitalize intellectual functions and reduce anxiety. (Bacosides are also found in Brain Wave Plus.)

JARSIN 300 OR 750 BY LICHTWER PHARMA

Without question, this is one of the best St. John's wort products on the market. There have been dozens of controlled clinical trials that demonstrate that St. John's wort is effective as a mood stabilizer. It also alleviates symptoms of mild to moderate depression, improves stress tolerance, overall mental performance, and immune function. St. John's wort has also been found to be helpful in controlling food cravings, improving energy, and dispelling those annoying "winter blues." A word of caution: don't take St. John's wort if you are taking MAO inhibitors or SSRIs, such as Prozac, Paxil, or Zoloft.

NEUHERIN BY ECOLOGICAL FORMULAS

This is a potent, compact brain booster containing acetyl-L-carnitine, ginkgo extract, and alithiamine (a fast-acting form of the vitamin thiamine). It's simply formulated for a "lite" hit of brain support.

COGNITEX BY LIFE EXTENSION

This is a highly sophisticated formulation that could only add to one's *optimal performance war chest*. It includes glyceryl phosphorylcholine, which acts as a choline donor and has been shown, for instance, to produce superior results in patients with dementia. It also prevents the age-related loss of cholinergic receptors, as well as the loss of neural tissue in the cerebellum (a large portion of the brain that coordinates voluntary movements, posture, and balance). Cognitex is a rich, well-developed product that improves brain function and provides potent brain-boosting nutrients designed to correct molecular damage that aging inflicts on brain cells.

Fat Burning and Metabolic Enhancement

There is no easy way to put this list together; there are simply too many products on the market for it to be an exhaustive compilation. The products listed below, by themselves and in combination, have been shown to produce maximum results. As always, be sure to consult with your health provider before taking any of these products.

Many of them contain thermogenic agents that are known for their effectiveness in releasing stored fat, especially when the "releasing mechanisms" aren't working well on their own. "Thermogenics" is a term that refers to anything that stimulates the burning of fat. Many people think being overweight is due to a sluggish metabolism. However, many people struggling with unwanted fat actually have quite adequate resting metabolic rates. The problem may be a breakdown in any one of the regulatory elements in the *group of dynamics* (see chapter 4) that determine how much you weigh, and how much of that weight will be in fat.

Even with their thermogenic agents, none of these products are going to magically burn away the unwanted pounds. In fact, some may actually produce unpleasant side effects, from heightened anxiety to sleeplessness.

That said, however, the products listed below are effective metabolism enhancers *when used in conjunction with the Paleotech Diet and Paleofitness guidelines*. Many contain ephedra, a controversial substance that, as discussed in chapter 4, has been deemed by the FDA to be safe and effective in doses of up to 90 milligrams a day.

When you combine the three nutrient elements of caffeine, ephedrine, and salicin, you create a "stack," a formula in which the impact of its parts produces a stronger effect than any one nutrient by itself. You'll probably need to do some experimentation in this area to determine which of these products, alone and/or in combination, work best for you. With the proper understanding of how they work, you can "stack" them even further to produce *synergy*.

XENADRINE BY CYTODENE TECHNOLOGIES

This is a hard-core fat burner. It contains thermogenic herbs, including ephedra. It also contains mood brighteners and energy stimulants, such as acetyl-L-carnitine and DMAE. It has a rapid intense effect; you can feel it working within the first hour. As with many of these products, safety precautions are on the label.

THERMICORE CRT BY MET-Rx

This is a great "smooth" fat burner. Less intense than Xenadrine, it is designed to be a time-release thermogenic. It includes green tea extract and is an exceptional product for anyone interested in a slower absorption curve of the ingredients.

TRIPHETAMINE BY PHARMALOGIC

From the mind and lab of Dr. Jim Jamieson, master pharmacologist, creator of the best over-the-counter growth hormone–releasing product, ProhGH, comes an equally powerful and effective fat burner. Triphetamine is designed to decrease appetite, burn body fat, eliminate water retention, and inhibit the conversion of carbohydrates to fat. It also includes several brain boosters. Many people who are overweight also complain of a lack of energy and a resultant lack of enthusiasm for exercise. This product often improves energy dramatically and can be useful in making you feel energetic enough to participate in a fitness program.

CLA (CONJUGATED LINOLEIC ACID)
BY LIFE EXTENSION, TWINLABS

CLA is a fatty acid found in foods and a main component of red meat that—get this—may prevent cancer. Further research has shown that aside from being a potent anticancer agent, it is an anticatabolic agent (meaning it protects against losing muscle), an immune stimulant, and, through a unique mechanism, *a fat-burning agent*.

CLA has become a popular supplement among fitness enthusiasts because of this last feature. It is a potent antioxidant that also lowers cholesterol and may be useful in a wide range of inflammatory disorders due to its ability to reduce an inflammatory eicosanoid known as PGE2.

Muscle Building and Power

These multifunctional products have great potential to build muscle, power, and endurance. Since you lose muscle and gain fat as you age, by the time you hit your seventies, you may lose 20 to 30 percent of the muscle mass you had in your twenties. These products, even in small amounts, will help you maintain your muscle mass, as long as you continue to exercise. Their effectiveness can also be amplified by stacking.

CREATINE MONOHYDRATE PRODUCTS BY EAS, TWINLABS, ET AL.
The term used to describe what creatine does is "cell volumizing," the process by which water molecules are pulled into the muscle cell, helping them look fuller and more pumped. This effect creates the necessary conditions for muscle growth. Creatine is one of the most popular supplements in bodybuilding. It is a compound that is made in our bodies and converted to an energy compound in the muscles known as creatine phosphate. Creatine helps increase muscle size and strength, and prevents the muscle tissue breakdown that can occur due to strenuous exercise. Used as a supplement, it can lead to dramatic increases in muscle mass. The theory goes that by loading up on creatine (thus increasing stores in the body), we can perform an exercise with greater intensity before reaching failure, thus allowing for significant gains in strength.

HMB BY EAS, TWINLABS, ET AL.

This product is like creatine junior. It is, however, an exceptional cell volumizer on its own, although many formulations combine both HMB and creatine. It's a natural substance also made by the human body, an amino acid that prevents muscle breakdown, boosts strength levels, and increases muscle size. A study examining the effects that HMB had on adults over sixty-five who trained with weights discovered it helped them achieve better results in a shorter period of time. Another study showed that women who exercised regularly while taking HMB gained more muscle strength and burned more fat.

EAS makes a great combination product called Betagen that I use and recommend as part of my muscle mass support program. It combines creatine monohydrate and HMB along with taurine and glutamine, which are also cell volumizers of a slightly lower order. Glutamine itself is exceptional for supporting both intestinal and immune function.

ZMA BY TWINLABS, ET AL.

ZMA is zinc monomethionine aspartate. It is often combined with magnesium aspartate. Its primary goal, like the other products in this category, is to boost strength levels, prevent muscle tissue breakdown, and enhance muscle size. It seems that ZMA does this using a different pathway than cell volumizers, as ZMA seems to exert a positive effect on natural anabolic hormones such as testosterone and GH (growth hormone).

A 1999 study done by Dr. Lorrie Brilla of Western Washington University, and presented to the American College of Sports Medicine, followed a group of football players who took ZMA for eight weeks. The ZMA group increased free testosterone levels by 43 percent more than the subjects who took a placebo. In addition, this group increased its muscle strength by 250 percent more than the placebo group.

A PROMISING MOLECULE

There are many products that show promise in this arena, including ribose, a molecule that is critical in the continuous production of ATP (the energy molecule), which gives our heart and muscles the energy they need to perform. Ribose is useful in increasing power for short periods of intense physical activity. It has been shown to enhance the rate at which ATP is replenished in the muscles, especially after demanding energy requirements. Excellent as a preworkout supplement.

OKG

This is a bond of the amino acid ornithine and alpha ketoglutarate, an "energy cycle" intermediate nutrient found in our bodies. This is a great product to stack with others in this category and offers a wide range of muscle and strength building properties. It also increases growth hormone and supports fat loss.

Anti-Aging Hormone Support: Growth Hormone Releasers; Secretagogues

A secretagogue is a nutraceutical combination of peptides, vitamins, pharmaceutical sugars (a nutrient that enables better absorption of the secretagogues), and amino acids that stimulates the pituitary gland to secrete growth hormone. There are two top-quality secretagogues that I recommend, the creations of the pharmacologist James Jamieson. I'll talk more specifically about growth hormone replacement therapy in the section on reversing aging (chapter 9). These products are additional pieces of your personal High-Tech program. They are aspects of constructing better health piece by piece; they are not *the ultimate solution to aging*.

So now let's look at the secretagogues and what they can do for you.

AN ASIDE ON SUCCESSFUL ADAPTATION AND AGING

It is important to note that successful aging is an *emergent phenomenon*. A flower is an emergent phenomenon; it is the sum total of all the energy generated by the plant to create it. Living to a vigorous old age is like a game of Monopoly. It's a function of getting your game piece in the right locations, along with some luck from tossing your dice, and a modicum of cunning. Now, if you are lucky enough, have a strategy, play your cards right, and learn from past mistakes, you may "emerge" a winner.

If you think you can control your aging by taking an elixir, you're reducing all the elements that must be considered down to some bottom line that simply does not exist. In fact, George Vaillant, professor of psychiatry at Harvard Medical School and director of the Study of Adult Development at Harvard University, is conducting an ongoing sixty-year study on successful aging. In one of the single most fascinating research studies ever conducted, successful aging can be sufficiently predicted by how well one scores inside of a "study model" influenced by the work of psychoanalyst Erik H. Erickson. In addition, the study model includes how well someone successfully adapts to life by comparing both protective factors (like good nutrition and fitness) before the age of fifty and risk factors, also before the age of fifty. Participants also fill out biennial questionnaires. The results of what came to be known as the "Study of Adult Development" are astounding: yes, good health is required, but so is the cultivation of the "psychobiological" dynamics, such as career identification (identified by the level of contentment), commitment (attachment to your work), and competence (pride in your work). These are factors that affect life expectancy and physical efficiency as we age.

PROHGH SPORT FOR MEN AND PROHGH SPORT FOR WOMEN BY PHARMALOGIC

This is the primary over-the-counter product that can be taken orally to stimulate the natural secretion of growth hormone (GH). Growth hormone exerts its effect on almost all tissues of the body. As we age, natural production of growth hormone decreases, and we actually become less sensitive to it at our receptor sites. As you'll find out in a later chapter, growth hormone can be injected. If you're interested in improving your GH levels without using injections, ProhGH is the way to go.

Growth hormone is naturally produced in the pituitary gland, located at the base of the brain. In your twenties you may "release" GH about twelve times a day during a twenty-four-hour period. After the age of thirty, the number and intensity of "releases" drop 14 percent for every decade you're alive. Some elderly people don't release any detectable GH at all. As you age and your GH drops, you may experience effects like:

- reduced lean body mass

- reduced skeletal mass

- decrease in exercise performance abilities

- increased abdominal and visceral fat

- elevated cholesterol

- thin skin

- decreased nail and hair growth

- reduced energy

- depression

Get the point . . . ?

The ProhGH products are elegantly designed to provide consistent and significant GH release while improving delivery to and absorption at the proper receptor sites. These products have been demonstrated to improve:

- muscle strength

- muscle size

- fat reduction

- exercise tolerance and endurance

- skin texture

- wrinkle reduction

- mental competence

The male version has an added element of the herb tribulus terrestris, a plant-based phytogenin. This is a compound that may naturally "turn on" testosterone production. The women's version contains natural isoflavones from soy, added to support female hormonal health.

TESTRON BY NUTRACEUTICS

An example of a nutraceutical that will provide native hormone support (similar to human testosterone in its makeup, also referred to as androgenic or androgen support) for the male is Testron. If you are looking for a natural alternative to male hormone replacement therapy, there are numerous products available on the market. Many of them are hawked on radio and in magazines promising renewed virility. The formulations usually include an herb known as yohimbe, a central nervous stimulant that increases

HGH (also known as somatotropin) is one of several hormones like testosterone, estrogen, progesterone, and DHEA that decline with age. Somatotropin, when brought back to acceptable levels, not only inhibits biological aging but significantly reverses many of its effects. Some of the other hormones can be replaced through the use of nutraceuticals and/or direct hormone replacement from your doctor.

arousal. They may include testosterone precursors such as androsteniadine. Most of these products are simply crude. I prefer Testron, which is what is called an adaptagen formula, consisting of six different enzyme-activated herbs, phytochemicals, and glandular extracts, which produce the *synergy* for optimal nonmedical testosterone support.

PROGESTA KEY CREAM BY UNI KEY

When it comes to female hormone support, there are multitudes of products available, and almost as much misinformation. We'll talk about menopause and perimenopause more in chapter 14. However, one of the best things you can do if you're a perimenopausal or menopausal woman is to get a copy of *Before the Change*, by Ann Louise Gittleman, which contains all the information you need to support your body properly throughout the years before and up to menopause.

How do you know if you're perimenopausal? If you're thirty-five or older, you've entered a period of time called the *climacteric*, which encompasses the hormonal changes that occur between the ages of thirty-five and sixty. The impact of perimenopause on the female body, especially if you don't know what's going on—can affect you in many ways, from your sex drive to your mental state. One of the reasons it affects some women so strongly is that their hormones (specifically estrogen and progesterone) are changing, and they *don't know it!* An essential nutraceutical, a native (similar to human progesterone in its makeup) and natural progesterone cream that I recommend for female hormone support is Progesta Key Cream. Progesterone creams can balance out estrogen-dominant symptoms during the years of perimenopause, such as decreased sex drive, depression, fatigue, irritability, bloating, fat gain, and weak thyroid function.

PROESTRON BY NUTRACEUTICS

If you are considering hormone replacement therapy (HRT), you may want to discuss this alternative with your doctor. ProEstron is derived from botanical sources, designed to target advancing menopausal symptoms.

DHEA is a hormone produced by the adrenal glands. This hormone also decreases as we age. At age eighty we produce only 10 to 20 percent of the DHEA we pumped out in our twenties. Its influence is global, affecting everything from how well our immune system performs to our level of mental function. DHEA is a benchmark of aging and a biomarker for longevity as measured in blood. Studies suggest that people with high DHEA levels live longer and have less heart disease and cancer. It increases estrogen production in women and testosterone in men to levels found in younger people. Its managed use can proffer multiple benefits in many health categories. DHEA:

- protects against bacterial and viral infections

- has an inhibitory effect on endotoxins (poisons contained in the cell walls of some bacteria) in our blood

- protects against diabetic damage

- has an antiobesity effect

- protects against arteriosclerosis

- is useful in the treatment of dementia and Alzheimer's

- may impact cognition, memory, and learning

The best way to incorporate DHEA and its "newer" version, 7-KETO, is to get either blood or salivary testing done (see functional assessment, page 244), and if levels are low, discuss the dosage with your healthcare provider.

It's important to note that proper testing and then proper hormone application can be very effective in preventing degenerative disease while improving physical and emotional health in both men and women. In many instances, doctors are quick to prescribe prescription drugs without testing and adjusting hormone levels with natural products. Many of the problems we face as we age, from abdominal weight gain to depression, could be eliminated without these drugs. For instance, there are well over two thousand published studies on DHEA demonstrating its role in improving neurological function, immune function, stress disorders, hormonal modulation, and many diseases associated with normal aging. Even with this body of evidence, doctors do not often test for DHEA levels; this might be a subject you want to bring up as part of taking charge of your own Healthy High-Tech Body program.

HORMONE REPLACEMENT THERAPY It's extremely important for women to explore many options before making HRT decisions. These supplements can be effective options for a High-Tech Body program. Be sure to read chapter 14 to find out about what's going on in your body, as well as chapter 10 to learn what kinds of tests you and your doctor can do to measure the changing landscape of your hormones. The only way to make appropriate decisions for your personal health is to gather as much knowledge as possible and weigh your options carefully.

The Longevity Nutrients You Must Have

This section began with some of the causes of aging, categories by which the human body physically succumbs to the disease of aging. No one has yet found the product(s) that will enable us to live forever. However, we can continue to exert control over how rapidly any one of these categories expands its territory in our bodies. The following list is made up of differing longevity nutrients; some are antioxidants, some are not, some blend nutrients that target and inhibit the expansion of one or more of these categories (nutrients that are active in a multitude of ways, in many organs and tissues at once, are called *pluripotent*). The following are some of the most effective longevity nutrients available today:

SUPER CARNOSINE CAPS BY LIFE EXTENSION

Carnosine is the epitome of longevity nutrients; it combats aging in a multitude of ways. It is a potent antioxidant and an antiglycation agent; it quenches aldehyde (a neurotoxin); it chelates harmful metals in our bodies; it converts senescent (aging) cells into juvenile ones; it prevents neurological degeneration and muscle atrophy; and it prevents cross-linking of collagen in our cells (a chemical reaction between free radicals and protein molecules) and in the lens of the eye. All of these factors accelerate the aging process and remote degenerative disease.

This product is pluripotent and *pan*-active, which means it works everywhere in our bodies, including and especially in the brain. It appears to be essential in protecting the skin from damage, loss of elasticity, and wrinkling, due to its primary function as an antiglycation agent. Glycation is an aging process in which proteins react with sugars. This leads to a loss of tissue tone and resiliency along with organ system degeneration.

VITAMIN E BY LIFE EXTENSION, THORNE RESEARCH, METAGENICS

A large prevention trial conducted by the National Cancer Institute and the National Public Health Institute of Finland, consisting of 29,133 male smokers (as reported in the *Journal of the National Cancer Institute*, March 18, 1998), showed that fifty- to sixty-nine-year-old men who took 50 milligrams of alpha-tocopherol (a form of the antioxidant vitamin E) daily for five to eight years had 32 percent fewer diagnoses of prostate cancer and 41 percent fewer prostate cancer deaths compared with men who did not receive vitamin E.

Additional benefits of vitamin E have been exhaustively documented, from reducing the risk of Alzheimer's disease to lowering the risk of ischemic and coronary heart disease, preventing blood clotting and reducing the risk of certain cancers. The well-known Cambridge Heart Antioxidant Study (CHAOS) looked at forty thousand men who already had heart disease. The study found that 400 to 800 IUs of vitamin E kept their heart disease from getting worse and cut their risk of having a fatal heart attack by an amazing 77 percent.

Another age-related problem is deteriorating vision. A study reported in the 1996 *American Journal of Epidemiology* was conducted to determine the association between blood levels of vitamin E and the development of cataracts. The study looked at 410 men for three years and concluded *that the men with the lowest levels of vitamin E had a 3.7 times greater risk of cataract formation than those with the highest levels of vitamin E.*

Remember that as we age, our own internal antioxidant enzymes become less active. As a result, there's even more free-radical production, which leads to accelerated aging and the increased need for supplemental antioxidants.

THE RIGHT VITAMIN

Here's the High-Tech secret: you don't want just any vitamin E, you want a combination that includes two forms known as d-gamma-tocopherol and d-alpha-tocopherol. These are extremely bioactive forms of vitamin E and should constitute part of a well-designed supplement program.

ALOE SELTZER VITAMIN C BY NUTRACEUTICS

Where do you begin describing the hierarchy of benefits derived from vitamin C? It is pluripotent, essential to everything from the production of collagen (the tissue that holds us together) to reducing the inflammatory eicosanoids that damage our bodies. Its role in *strengthening* our immunity is richly documented, and it is this property of vitamin C that brings me to endorse this High-Tech secret, Aloe Seltzer C (as you might gather from its name, this is an effervescent form of vitamin C). It's made from the aloe vera cactus; more specifically, it has an added immune-enhancing extract of aloe known as Betamannin.

Vitamin C comes in many forms, from ester-C to buffered-C. This "C" is designed for *improved delivery*. Besides being a powerful antioxidant and immune enhancer, it is restorative, helping weakened adrenal systems perform better. It is another great mitigator of jet lag and can be stacked with proendorphins to improve energy.

Folic Acid, B_{12}, B_6, SAMe, and Trimethylglycine

A number of years ago I read of a doctor named Kilmer McCully, who had discovered a connection between heart disease and the accumulation of a toxic amino acid called homocysteine. For many years, his suggestion that the problem of accumulating homocysteine could be reduced by taking folic acid, as well as vitamins B_6 and B_{12}, was not taken seriously. Recently, however, studies have shown that elevated levels of homocysteine in the blood are linked to an increased risk of premature coronary artery disease, stroke, and thromboembolism (blood clots) *even among people with normal cholesterol*. Excess homocysteine does damage in the following ways:

1. It has a direct toxic effect that damages the inside lining of the arteries.

2. It causes LDL cholesterol (the "bad" kind) to oxidize.

3. It interferes with blood-clotting factors.

4. It interferes with a detoxifying process called methylation; this interference may be a major cause of aging.

There are a number of well-known risk factors that can be used to predict the likelihood of having a heart attack or stroke, among them such obvious things as cigarette smoking, lack of physical activity, and excess abdominal fat. Now we must add elevated homocysteine levels. Studies have shown that about 10 percent of heart attacks and strokes can be attributed to high levels of homocysteine—that's more than a hundred thousand deaths every year in the United States alone. Additional studies have confirmed that people with Alzheimer's-type dementia have elevated levels of homocysteine in their blood; it may then be that homocysteine is a biomarker for the development of Alzheimer's-type dementia. Anyone with a family history of heart disease, stroke, or Alzheimer's is at risk for elevated homocysteine. High homocysteine levels have also been linked to complications in diabetes, lupus, and other chronic illnesses. The best thing to do is get your blood levels measured. Normal ranges are 5 to 15 micromoles per liter of blood, although it seems that a level above 6.3 causes a steep, progressive risk of heart disease (*Circulation* magazine, November 15, 1995).

You can reduce homocysteine levels through two detoxification routes. The most common route is called the remethylation process, which requires folic acid, vitamin B_{12}, zinc, and a nutrient called trimethylglycine (TMG). The second pathway, called transsulfuration, is dependent on vitamin B_6. Lowering homocysteine has been proven to reduce the risk of adverse cardiovascular events. At the very least, you should be tested for homocysteine levels and take folic acid to reduce high levels.

SAMe

One of the benefits of taking TMG to reduce homocysteine is that TMG converts homocysteine to SAMe, or s-adenosylmethione. SAMe is an amino acid derivative normally found in the body. It has been used as an antidepressant in Europe for years; a recent study from the University of Rome showed that SAMe is as effective as some conventional antidepressants. It has almost no side effects (although it should not be taken in combination with other antidepressants) and is believed to be one of the safest, most effective antidepressants in the world. It is also thought to offer significant support for liver function and has been found to protect against osteoarthritis and heart disease.

Joints, Muscles, and Ligaments

GLUCOSAMINE/CHONDROITIN

Diseases of the joints have been around for millions of years. Paleontologists have even found that some bones from dinosaurs that lived over a hundred million years ago displayed evidence of arthritis. Evidence of arthritis has been found in Egyptian mummies and in remains of prehistoric man.

Our joints are held together by cartilage, a gel-like substance that acts as a shock absorber for our bones. Cartilage is made of collagen and glycosaminoglycan molecules. Collagen and glycosaminoglycan are produced by special cells, called chondrocytes, in the cartilage. Glucosamine, which is naturally produced in the body, stimulates the manufacture of glycosaminoglycan. The inability to produce glucosamine may be a leading factor in the development of osteoarthritis.

Glucosamine is another supplement that has been used extensively in Europe for many years. Recently, it has been found that chondroitin sulfate, a glycosaminoglycan, can be used in combination with glucosamine to reduce joint pain and cartilage damage and even reverse osteoarthritis.

MSM

MSM is an abbreviation of methylsulfonylmethane, a form of sulfur that is found naturally in fresh fruits, vegetables, and many other foods. Unfortunately, food processing and soil depletion have dramatically decreased our dietary sulfur supply. Sulfur is a fundamental building material of our bodies and is essential to our survival. Sulfur is often referred to as the "beauty mineral," because it softens tissue and keeps cells from becoming rigid. Without enough sulfur, cells become thin and tough, trapping toxins in and oxygen and nutrients out. Sulfur is used by the body to form crucial proteins and amino acids.

MSM has an incredibly wide array of benefits:

- increased oxygenation, resulting in higher energy and better detoxification

- improved skin, hair, and nails

- increased blood circulation

- reduced joint pain and stiffness

- reduced inflammation

- relief from asthma

- increased mental alertness

- controls acidity in stomach and ulcers

- rehabilitates intestinal tract lining

- improved digestion and absorption of nutrients

This chapter may seem a bit overwhelming. So many supplements, so little time . . . Not to mention the fact that there are new discoveries every day. You can't—and shouldn't—take everything. You might want to take some of these supplements for general Healthy High-Tech maintenance. On the other hand, if you're having problems in specific areas, take the appropriate supplements listed here until those problems are solved. Don't take any of these products blindly. There are many books available that go into great detail about supplements, and there's an incredible amount of information on the Internet. Do your homework and find the supplements that will keep you functioning most efficiently toward your goal of High-Tech health.

6 Detoxification

Getting the euphoria up
by getting the toxins out

The upside of living in the modern world is the incredible advantage science and technology have given us in staying healthy and living longer. We are learning more every day about how our bodies function and what we can do to keep them functioning most efficiently. In the last four chapters we've seen how we can use food, exercise, and supplementation to rev up that efficiency almost to its peak.

If you want to eliminate the "almost" and keep your body running in top Healthy High-Tech form, there is one more important step you need to consider: detoxification.

Detoxification is the metabolic process by which toxins—poisonous compounds in the body—are changed into less toxic or more easily excretable substances. It is the method by which the body cleanses itself of those substances that, left alone, would do us harm.

Every machine needs to be cleaned out every once in a while. You change the oil in your car so that the engine can run more efficiently. You change the filter in your air conditioner. You keep dust away from your computer. You even clean the heads on your VCR in order to make it last longer and play better. You're constantly removing the gunk that impairs the functionality of the machines that make your life easier.

Toxins are your body's gunk, and they do damage in several ways. They are poisonous to the cells themselves, they disrupt the metabolism of cells, or they interfere with digestion. The consequences of toxins are wide-ranging. They include:

- allergies

- Alzheimer's disease

- bad breath

- bowel problems

- cardiovascular problems

- depression

- fatigue

- gastrointestinal tract irregularities

- headache

- irritability

- muscle and joint pain

- Parkinson's disease

- PMS

And, to put it bluntly, the more toxic we are, the faster we age.

Toxins, Toxins Everywhere

We live in a toxic world. There are toxins everywhere: in the air we breathe, the water we drink, the food we eat. They come from pesticides and additives and bus fumes and chemicals and industrial waste. They're in coffee and alcohol and tobacco. The drugs we've taken over the years—legal and illegal, over-the-counter and prescription—leave toxic residue.

Not all toxins are man-made, however. Toxins are found everywhere in nature as well. Many plants are loaded with chemicals they use as defense mechanisms. Since plants can't run from predators, they use these harmful chemicals to protect themselves from plant-eating microbes and insects. Not all plants contain toxins, of course, and some contain toxins only in their leaves or seeds. (Think of apricots, for instance. The fruit is delicious and healthy, while the seed [or pit] contains cyanide, which is toxic. That's probably because the species can survive only if the reproductive seed is protected.)

And, as if plant-based poisons were not enough, the human body even produces its own toxins. These are the waste products of our metabolism and are called endogenous toxins. Then there are the bacteria, some healthy and some unhealthy, that live in our intestinal tract. When there are too many unhealthy bacteria, they release toxic by-products into our system, which contribute to many diseases and general feelings of ill health.

Although the body has been designed with several built-in filtration systems, these systems cannot always handle the overload of today's toxic environments. In many instances, these toxic residues are fat soluble; that is, they remain behind in our tissues and our bodies don't have the capacity to remove or reduce them in a timely manner.

"Natural" Detoxification: The Body Takes Care of Itself

Since human beings don't have a filtration system that we can take out and clean periodically, we have to find ways of cleaning out the system from within. If we don't, we can severely damage the efficient functioning of the bodies we try so hard to maintain through diet, exercise, and supplementation.

Our bodies have several different filtering systems of our own. These systems include:

Intestines In their healthy state, the intestines help get rid of toxins through regular bowel movements, by eliminating unhealthy microorganisms, and by providing a strong barrier against leakage into the blood system.

Kidneys The kidneys' main purpose is to provide the major escape route for toxins, through the urine.

Skin We sweat through the pores in our skin. Sweat is an excellent system for releasing many of the toxins in our bodies, which is one of the reasons we smell so bad after a good sweaty workout.

Fat Although fat is not a filtering system per se, the reduction of fat helps eliminate toxins. Excess toxins often deposit themselves into fat cells, where they tend to stay, and the only way to get rid of those toxins is to get rid of the excess fat—in other words, lose weight.

Liver The liver filters out and transforms toxins that have entered the bloodstream into harmless substances that can be excreted in the urine.

Much of the detoxification that goes on in the body happens in the liver, which is the base of the process called biotransformation: taking harmful chemicals in the body and transforming them into substances that can be either easily absorbed or excreted. Biotransformation is a two-phase process.

In Phase 1, a "super family" of enzymes, called the cytochrome P450 system, transforms the toxins into metabolites. In Phase 2, these metabolites are further transformed so that they can be eliminated in the urine, feces, or sweat.

Sometimes, however, the transformation is incomplete; the metabolites get stuck in their Phase 1 form and remain toxic (this process is called bioactivation).

This is why you sometimes feel worse during the detoxification process; until it's complete, you may be producing even more toxins than before. Not only that, the metabolites that are formed then produce free radicals. A free radical is an oxygen molecule with an odd number of electrons in the outer ring of one of its atoms. Free radicals grab on to healthy cells and try to "steal" their electrons. These free radicals are what do us harm.

When our bodies suffer from toxic overload, we need to help our natural detoxification systems along. Some animals do this instinctively. For instance, chimpanzees often eat clay, which is thought to have detoxifying abilities, from termite mounds and other sources. And Indians in both North and South America have been known to prepare some foods with clay to absorb some of their harmful substances and make them safe for consumption.

THE HUMAN ADVANTAGE In her book *The Primal Feast*, Susan Allport notes that although animals such as chimps have found natural methods of detoxification, humans are the ". . . only cooks on the planet. We tend to think of cooking as a way of making food taste better, but it has an even more important use. It is, first and foremost, a way of overcoming plant defenses, a way of making foods that would otherwise be toxic or indigestible completely edible." This is one of the reasons for the survival of the human species.

We have also survived by creating new versions of plants that are free of their original toxic substances, foods such as yams, potatoes, cucumbers, and watermelons. That makes them easier for humans to consume. However, it also makes them easier for microbes and insects to consume; so man developed pesticides to keep the insects away. Those pesticides are often more toxic than the original substances we were trying to eliminate. Talk about a catch-22!

Allport also notes another method humans created to help natural detoxification—the use of spices. People often wonder why inhabitants of the hottest countries often eat the spiciest foods. Researchers now believe that it is because many spices, including allspice, cinnamon, oregano, cayenne, mustard, and garlic, have ". . . powerful antibacterial and antifungal effects. All are capable of killing or suppressing seventy-five to one hundred percent of the bacteria and fungi that commonly contaminate and spoil foods." This means that we have learned to detoxify some substances before they even enter our bodies.

The Nutritional Approach
to Detoxification

What does nutrition have to do with detoxification? Not too long ago, it was thought that water and juice fasts were the way to clear toxins out of the body. But a study published in the *Annual Review of Nutrition* in 1991 showed that fasting actually decreases your protection against free radicals. It also showed that efficient functioning of the cytochrome P450 system requires adequate dietary protein; prolonged fasting weakens muscles and various organs because of protein losses and a slowing of metabolic activity. Furthermore, it appears that a high carbohydrate intake reduces the ability of the P450 enzymes to work effectively. So the best way to bolster your natural detoxification system is to follow the Paleotech Diet, consuming a relatively high amount of protein and fewer carbohydrates.

Here are some dietary guidelines for efficient detoxification:

Include protein at every meal Protein is rich in a detoxifying enzyme called glutathione (also known as GSH), which Dr. Mitchell Gaynor (author of *Dr. Gaynor's Cancer Prevention Program*) calls "the most abundant antioxidant in the human body and perhaps the most important." Including a daily dose of at least 500 milligrams of vitamin C helps the body manufacture glutathione from proteins. (Glutathione is also found in some fruits and vegetables, including grapefruit, oranges, strawberries, tomatoes, cantaloupe, watermelon, potatoes, broccoli, spinach, asparagus, acorn squash, and zucchini.)

Be sure to get enough fiber This is the reason for those six servings of fiber-rich fruits and vegetables, especially green leafy vegetables, such as spinach, watercress, lettuces (including mesclun), and a wide variety of sprouts. Add in vegetables like asparagus, peapods, tomatoes, carrots, zucchini, peppers, radishes, and cucumbers, and cooked cruciferous vegetables, such as broccoli, kale, cauliflower, cabbage, and Brussels sprouts. Don't forget fruits, such as apples and berries.

Add in antioxidants Red, yellow, and green vegetables are high in antioxidants. So are raw seeds and nuts.

Drink six to eight glasses of water a day Simply drinking water flushes out many of the body's impurities.

Increase omega-3 fatty acids Omega-3 fatty acids increase the Phase 2 enzyme activity in the body. Fish like salmon, sardines, halibut, tuna, mackerel, bass, swordfish, mahi-mahi, cod, trout, and shellfish like crab and shrimp are high in omega-3 fatty acids, as are olive oil, fish oil, flaxseed oil, and many nuts and seeds.

Avoid refined carbohydrates Sugar and processed flours have been shown to slow down the activity of P450 (Phase 1) enzymes, thus inhibiting the body's ability to rid itself of harmful toxins.

The High-Tech Approach to Detoxification

Our bodies' own detoxification processes take care of most of the endogenous toxins—by-products of our own metabolism—that build up in our systems. But living in our High-Tech world, we also have to deal with exogenous toxins: molecular structures that enter the body from the environment. These exogenous toxins, all the pollutants that man has created, are the burden of the nonnatural world. It's impossible to avoid these toxins, no matter how careful we are.

Some people are affected by these toxins more than others. Two people may live near the same chemical plant. One may suffer constant complaint and discomfort, while the other doesn't seem to be bothered at all. In extreme circumstances, there are people who have what we now call "environmental illness," people who seem to be allergic to just about everything around them.

There are several categories of exogenous toxins we deal with every day:

- **Carcinogens:** substances known to cause cancer, such as tobacco.

- **Neurotoxins (also known as excitotoxins):** substances added to foods and beverages that causes undue nerve stimulation, such as caffeine, MSG, and artificial sweeteners.

- **Hormone disruptors:** chemicals from outside the body that can interfere with the development or functioning of body systems, such as chemical waste and petrochemical plastic by-products.

These are compounds that disrupt metabolic efficiency. They can affect muscles, joints, cardiovascular function, and produce immune disorders. If you want to stop the disruption of that efficiency, if you want to bring your body up to its High-Tech potential, you must remove these toxic substances. While the preceding nutritional guidelines are a great start, they are not enough.

In this High-Tech, highly toxic world, we need some more advanced methods of cleansing and detoxifying our bodies.

The High-Tech Detox Solutions

Let's do a quick recap: The human body uses the different processes of detoxification, a complex series of reactions to rid itself of toxins whose chronic presence may have damaging effects on tissues and lead to imbalances and functional disruption along many different physical pathways. Impairing or overburdening the detoxification system can have dire consequences for us. Internal toxic accumulation of anything from petrochemical hydrocarbons, drugs of all kinds, bacterial by-products, and other complex and weird molecules has been shown to contribute and be intimately related to such adverse health conditions as Parkinson's disease, certain types of cancers, fibromyalgia, and chronic fatigue syndrome. Clearly, supporting your own Phase 1 and Phase 2 detoxification pathways is critical. Many people find that following a well-thought-out detoxification regimen (or what I like to call a clearing program) is of great benefit—not only because it relieves various "annoying" symptoms, but because it provides a *return of well-being that has oftentimes simply been missing!*

There are two key ways to support your own detoxification *and find yourself feeling better than you have in years.* Of course, before embarking on any such program, you must discuss it with your doctor or healthcare practitioner, just to be sure it doesn't interfere with any medications you are taking or medical problems you may be experiencing.

The clearing programs that I recommend to my clients and use myself come from the protocols defined by the field of Functional Medicine, which I consider the true medicine of the twenty-first century (see chapter 10, "Diagnostics").

Your Home Detox Program: Get the Euphoria Up and the Toxins Out

What is most amazing about detoxification is that you can actually feel an immediate difference. Even if you didn't know you were feeling poorly, complete a detoxification program and you'll feel much better. Speak to anyone who has detoxed—whether through a hard-core cleansing, or just a sauna after a good workout at the gym—and you can see the improvement in their mood and overall well-being. Some people have even reported feelings of euphoria. If you consistently take care of yourself according to the guidelines of detoxification, you'll begin to accumulate good feelings, not toxins. Detoxification can bring certain relief from physical discomfort, a drop in inflammation, improved sleeping, heightened relaxation, and clarity of mind.

The Sauna: Turning Up the Heat

Variously referred to as biotoxic reduction therapy, hyperthermic detoxification, or just plain sauna therapy, this method of detoxification has been used for centuries by cultures around the world for detoxification and overall well-being. According to current nutritional, medical and biomedical literature, detoxification is capable of significantly reducing and/or eliminating stored toxic residue. It has been proven to be scientifically safe, according to Dr. David Schnara (science adviser to the Environmental Protection Agency). Countless studies (dating back through several decades and confirmed by organizations as far ranging as the Royal Swedish Academy of Sciences, the Mt. Sinai School of Medicine, and the World Health Organization) have shown the impact of saunas on unburdening and clearing the human body of such deadly compounds as PCBs, organohalides, and PCPs. Saunas have also been shown to be very effective in removing occupational and environmental chemical residue.

As you sweat, toxins are secreted from where they're stored: your skin, your organs, and your fat tissue. Measurable amounts of metabolic waste products with unfamiliar names, such as n-alkanes, paraffinic hydrocarbons, and amphetamine metabolites, are secreted. That's a good thing—you don't want these waste products sitting in your body, busily *bioaccumulating and bioaltering you.*

The Slow Melt

Detoxification doesn't mean you have to go into a sauna and roast. You should never take an extended sauna (more than forty-five minutes) unless you are being medically supervised. The most effective method is the "cool sauna," or what I like to call the "slow melt." The point is to heat your fat sufficiently so that the toxins stored within it are released through your sweat glands. A good sauna can improve circulation, reduce bloating and edema, and help clear your complexion. It also promotes the release of endorphins in the brain (chemical neurotransmitters responsible for the "runner's high"), which no doubt accounts for the euphoria many people experience.

It also turns out that the sauna increases circulation on the surface of our tissues (improving our appearance) and also goes deep within the tissues, improving both blood-fat levels and microcirculation to the brain, which consequently improves brain function. A 1982 study involving 103 people showed, after a sauna, a mean increase in the Wechsler Intelligence Scale IQ of 6.7 points along with improvements in a broad range of psychological test scores.

High-Tech Saunas

Although going to your local health club for a sauna is very effective, there is a new type of sauna available that you can install in your home. It is called an infrared sauna. The infrared thermal heat penetrates deep into the body, inducing up to two or three times the volume of sweat of a traditional hot stone sauna. There is deeper penetration of the infrared rays (over 1.5 inches more) into the skin, stimulating deep tissue and internal organs more effectively. These are "cool" saunas, operating at a range of 110 to 130 degrees, with greater efficacy than a standard sauna. There are now several companies in America producing infrared sauna devices, which you can find in the resource section of this book.

In the absence of radiant heat saunas, any sauna will suffice. The optimal heat exposure in a standard sauna for detoxing purposes (say at your local fitness club) often varies between 150 and 200 degrees. The tolerance to both heat and time exposure varies from person to person, with a general time of about twenty to thirty minutes in "the box," which should be alternated with periods of cooling down.

Some people have to get out of the sauna every five to ten minutes, cool off, and go back in. You may even want to take a cold shower during the cooldown. In many countries, it is standard practice to sauna for a short time, then take a cold plunge (into a cold pool or even outside into the snow), and then return to the sauna.

The Niacin Tweak

If you want to help your sauna along in the process of removing toxins, you may want to use niacin (vitamin B_3), before entering the sauna. Vitamin B_3 is a potent mobilizer of fat and the toxins embedded in fat. This vitanutrient is a powerful vasodilator: as it increases blood flow to the periphery of your skin, it can produce a strong flushing sensation. It has broad uses and applications. There are a number of protocols where it is used to reduce cholesterol and keep a "sticky" damaging blood protein, lipoprotein (a), from damaging your arteries. In this case, niacin potentiates the effects of the sauna.

However, the use of niacin for detoxification purposes should be carefully monitored by a clinician familiar with its use and application. The recommended dosage is 50 to 300 milligrams about ten to fifteen minutes before entering the sauna. This is not something that should be done before every sauna; you can use it three or four times a year for a more intense detoxification. The effects of the niacin can last anywhere from fifteen minutes to an hour, but you can decrease the flushing faster by consuming more water.

The Power Sauna

There are spas and clinics that offer comprehensive sauna programs. They are always done under medical supervision and involve lengthy saunas (lasting anywhere from one to three hours), taken every day for a week. In these programs, great care must be taken to avoid dehydration and heat exhaustion.

So, there are three ways to sauna:

1 As a weekly addition to your personal care, after exercise.

2 Seasonally, as part of a lengthier detoxification program. That would include a sauna of a half hour to forty-five minutes, four or five times within one week.

3 As part of a medically supervised program at a *comprehensive cleansing facility*, where a comprehensive sauna detoxification program is offered.

There are basic rules that must be followed, no matter which sauna protocol you choose:

- Drink plenty of water during a sauna detox.

- Use an electrolyte replacement drink, such as Gatorade, during and after the sauna.

- Always build up your tolerance. Start with five minutes of sauna and five minutes of cooldown, then increase your times slowly.

- Sauna after exercise for a more effective cleansing.

- A detox isn't a race; do a few saunas a week to begin with; get the feel for it and build up your time slowly.

- For a lifetime of "clearing" do a sauna two to three times a week for a half hour to forty-five minutes with breaks and fluid replacement.

Ultraclear and Liver Resuscitation: The Second Leg of High-Tech Detoxification

I started conducting my own clearing programs almost twenty-five years ago. As I made changes in my lifestyle, transitioning from a kid of the sixties into someone whose lifestyle would define his future, there were a number of significant "eureka moments" along the way. I suffered from chronic migraine headaches for a number of years, starting in the early 1970s. I pursued the conventional medical routes, but found no acceptable solution. The neurologist I worked with had recommended that I use Cafergot, a potent migraine drug, which I had no interest in using, mostly because my mother (a lifelong migraine headache sufferer) was addicted to it. I had seen her demolished by both the headaches and the accelerating abuse of painkillers.

Now here I was at the same threshold, getting these headaches and wondering if this was to be my destiny also. At that time, very few doctors (if any) were looking into the root causes of migraines. The question of whether diet or any lifestyle practices were in any way affecting my migraines *never* came up. The fact that I smoked a pack of cigarettes a day, didn't work out, and ate junk food all the time never showed up as factors that should be considered. I distinctly remember walking out of my doctor's office onto Park Avenue, bursting into tears at the thought of having no other option.

I remember thinking that somebody, somewhere, must be doing *something* about migraines; I didn't even know where to begin to look. In one of those "coincidental" moments of life, I wandered into a health food store and noticed a display of books. One of them was called *The Miracle of Fasting* by Paul Bragg. This book literally changed my life. I started juice fasting, water fasting, growing my own sprouts, going to the Russian-Turkish sauna baths in lower Manhattan, doing colonics. I gave up sugar, white flour, meat, and cigarettes. I started jogging and doing meditation *and never looked back.* My friends and family thought I'd lost my marbles, but guess what? Along the way, I lost the migraines—not to mention my depression and bleeding gums, my bloating, my physical discomfort, and my exhaustion.

Since then I've refined and evolved my work. Fasting gave way to clearing with the advent of a "functional food" powder in the late eighties called **Ultraclear,** and that changed everything again.

Ultraclear is a food-based powder product designed to be consumed in beverage form; it's made from rice-protein concentrate and intended to be used as part of a detoxification program. It supplanted fasting as a way to detoxify, along with the scientific research in clinical nutrition to support its use and effectiveness. It's used to help the liver perform its detoxifying functions with greater efficiency, especially in Phase 2 activity. It's jam-packed with phytonutrients and minerals to protect the liver and promote hepatic antioxidant activity. Because of its unique composition of protein (required to detoxify properly), essential fats in the form of medium chain triglycerides (MCT), and the right percentage of carbohydrates, it's a perfect meal replacement during a detoxifying program. In addition, it's rich in glutathione (a powerful antioxidant required by the liver to reduce and eliminate toxins) and glutathione precursor nutrients. As an antioxidant, glutathione may directly scavenge free radicals and is required for the processing and elimination of toxic metabolic by-products that our body manufactures.

An Ultraclear detoxification program should be monitored by a healthcare practitioner trained in its use. There is a well-detailed and planned program designed for its implementation called the **Step Approach**, a gradual detox program conducted over a period of time that can range from one to seven days. Another Ultraclear program, the **4R Program**, is designed to optimize colon and bowel performance and to really get your "metabolic house" in order. It is intended to reduce and eliminate foods that harm you; to clear out pathogens, bacteria, and/or parasites that shouldn't be in your gastrointestinal tract; then go on to repair and restore the health of your colon and liver. For more information on detoxification or the 4R Program, go to www.healthcomm.com, or contact a healthcare practitioner trained in the use of Ultraclear.

A Final Word . . .

There are many paths to detoxification. Many spas and resorts provide their own custom-designed programs, as do many different practitioners. I highly endorse detoxification; I only stress that it be done with proper guidance, especially if it's your first time. Nonetheless, detoxification is an important but often overlooked tool to starting you on your way to High-Tech health and beyond.

Pillar 3

Life Extension,
Life Enhancement

The purpose of achieving a Healthy High-Tech Body is not just to live longer. It is to live longer better. What good does it do to extend a person's life to 120 years if many of those years are spent in pain and infirmity? Therefore, you cannot talk about life extension without also talking about life enhancement.

The thing that concerns us most as we age is possible loss of our cognitive abilities. We have lived; let us not forget. The most frightening picture we have of our elder selves is a mental wanderer, far removed from the people and places we loved the most.

We have not yet learned to conquer diseases like Alzheimer's and Parkinson's, but there is much that we can do to halt their progress. The first chapter in this pillar, **"The Power Brain,"** explores some of those options for you. But its main focus is on maintaining and/or improving your current capabilities. The elements of achieving a Power Brain have been divided into two parts: Preservation and Enhancement.

Part 1, Preservation, lays out what you'll have to do to preserve the brain's structure and reduce cell damage, while part 2, Enhancement, contains information on "assisting" the brain's efficiency through the use of smart drugs and nootropics.

The next two chapters, on injectables and human growth hormone, will take you traveling across the ocean and back again for the latest anti-aging treatments available. First, to Europe for twenty-first-century refinements in live cell therapy, a treatment that's been used in Germany, Switzerland, and France for several decades. I'll take you with me as I travel to Clinique La Prairie to find out what it's all about. Then it's back to the States, to Cenegenics, the ultramodern, ultra-High-Tech anti-aging facility in Las Vegas, Nevada, that specializes in human growth hormone therapy.

You may not know much about either of these two effective, but controversial, anti-aging treatments. You will definitely be hearing more and more about them in the future; you could be one of the "first kids on the block" to understand just what they can (and cannot) do for you. It's the only way to make educated decisions about directions you may want to take in developing a Healthy High-Tech Body.

The more you understand about how your body functions, the better you can take care of it. That's why diagnostics are so important. There's a burgeoning movement in the health field that is just as concerned with keeping you well as it is with treating your illnesses. It's called Functional Medicine. And the basis of this new field is functional analysis: finding out how well all your systems are currently working so that any problems or deficiencies can be discovered before they turn into major disease states.

7 The Power Brain

What you need to stay mentally sharp and keep your brain in the game

A recent newsmagazine printed a cover article about how to improve your memory. In it, the reporter tried ginkgo biloba, which, he reported, upset his stomach. He took a few memory-enhancement courses, but couldn't really tell if they helped. And that's about as far as it went. How disappointing that in this day and age—on the brink of our High-Tech future—the magazine chose to reduce such a complex issue to a few bare-bones components.

Although the brain is the most complex and remarkable organ in our body, more of what we know about it has been discovered in the past fifty years than in the rest of human history. So we are still in the early stages of discovering how the brain functions and how we can help it work better. But there is a lot we do know about it.

Here are the basics: the brain is a grayish, wrinkled, jellylike mass that weighs about three pounds in most adults. It's made up of several different parts:

Brain stem This is the oldest part of our brain (in evolutionary terms). Located at the top of the spine, it governs basic activities like breathing, heart rate, and digestion.

Cerebellum Located directly behind the brain stem, it governs the body's movement through space and maintains muscle coordination.

Limbic system This segment of the brain is perched on top of the brain stem and controls body temperature, blood pressure, and blood sugar. It's also responsible for emotional reactions, such as the "fight-or-flight" response. Parts of the limbic system, including the **hippocampus** and **amygdala**, are associated with processing information and memory formation.

C e r e b r u m The cerebrum is split into two sections, the left and right hemispheres of the brain, joined by a bridge of nerve fibers. The left hemisphere generally controls analytical functions, such as understanding language, speaking, computing, and general cognitive functions. The right hemisphere manages nonverbal and imaginative processes, such as recognizing patterns, reconstructing melodies, and visualizing images. In many cases, however, studies have shown that each of the brain's hemispheres has the potential of processing any function when a particular brain area is damaged by injury or disease.

The two hemispheres are covered by "gray matter" that is about one-eighth of an inch thick. This is the cortex, and it is what makes us human. The cortex is divided into four different areas, or lobes: (1) **frontal**—involved in decision making and problem solving; (2) **parietal**—involved in the reception of sensory information; (3) **occipital**—associated with vision; and (4) **temporal**—associated with hearing and language.

How It Works

The brain works through a highly sensitive network of about a hundred billion microscopic nerve cells, or **neurons.** Each neuron is surrounded by branchlike **dendrites** and one long trunklike appendage called the **axon.** Here's what happens when neurons are stimulated: a dendrite receives an electrical impulse (traveling at about two hundred miles an hour) from a neighboring neuron. This impulse travels through the axon to the cell's nucleus. The impulse directs the nucleus to release chemicals called **neurotransmitters;** the neurotransmitters flow into the gap (or

synapse) between one cell and its neighbor. This, in turn, stimulates the neighbor's dendrites, and the process continues.

Individual brains are as different as fingerprints, and the precise manner in which a particular brain operates varies according to genetics, diet, lifestyle, substance abuse, etc.

Raising Cognitive Efficiency

To achieve a High-Tech Power Brain, you need to address the **three dynamics** involved in raising the efficiency of the brain by maintaining, elevating, and/or improving the:

- **general cognitive power of the brain**

- **information-processing capabilities of the brain**

- **structural integrity of the brain**

You want to maintain the brain's structures and functions, its "hardware" and "circuitry," its nutrient environment, cells, neurons, glands, and all the tissues that make up its structure. Its functions should be fluid and reliable, like the performance of a well-oiled and well-maintained vehicle. There are two areas of brain function that are of major concern for most people, especially as they age: *memory* and *intelligence*. Luckily, these two areas can not only be maintained as we age, but can be improved by following the High-Tech protocols suggested in this chapter.

About Memory

Memory is a fundamental cognitive process that allows us to acquire and retain information about the world and our experiences within it. There are three stages in how we form memories: encoding, storage, and retrieval. *Encoding* is processing an event or information as it comes to you, *storage* is creating a record of that event or information, and *retrieval* is being able to play that event or information back when you want or need it.

According to current psychological theory there is a difference between the following:

procedural memory—"remembering how"

declarative memory—"remembering that"

Remembering *how* to ride a bicycle is procedural; remembering *that* something with a seat on a metal frame with two wheels is a bicycle is declarative. Let's go further.

Declarative memory can be split into "semantic" and "episodic" memory. Remembering that my birthday is February 12 is semantic; remembering what I did last February 12 *on* my birthday is episodic. It appears that the most vulnerable form of memory is episodic.

About Intelligence

According to Encarta on-line encyclopedia, intelligence refers to "a general mental capability to reason, solve problems, think abstractly, learn and understand new material, and profit from past experience." However, it goes on to say that there is "no universally accepted definition of intelligence."

I can't tell you how to get more intelligent. None of the suggestions or supplements in this chapter will help you join MENSA. However, they can facilitate the maintenance of "smartness." It's all about making your particular smartness work better for you, perform more efficiently. How you then use that smartness is determined by many other variables, including diet, sleep, environment, and how you've been training yourself to use your smartness.

Staying mentally "sharp" and keeping your brain in the game turns out to be the effect of *coalescing processes*, many factors working together to protect the brain itself from the ravages of use, abuse, and aging. Following the Power Brain protocols will result in improved cognitive efficiency, which we could simply define as reliable mental faculties, reliable memory, and reliable intelligence. In other words, keeping your wits about you as long as possible.

There is an art to staying mentally sharp and competent; this art of cognitive enhancement is made up of the following components:

- optimal nutrition

- good levels of fitness

- the use of proper nutraceuticals

- the use of nootropics

- the use of anti-inflammatory drugs

- sensory motor exercises

- mental exercises

- having an "enriched" environment (one that includes many different stimuli)

If you practice the "art" of cognitive enhancement, you should have tangible, palpable results such as:

- increased alertness

- alleviation of depression

- increased ability to concentrate for longer periods of time

- improved verbal memory

- greater productivity

- a consistently higher level of mental performance

- improved overall health

- reduced risk factors for neurological illness

- reversal of decreased or declining mental abilities

- improvement in abilities to learn, memorize, and recall

- mood brightening and elevation

These results cannot be achieved without consistent and focused effort. Although this chapter contains information about *smart drugs* available for your use today, cognitive enhancement does not happen automatically through some quick chemical fix. These chemicals can help, but only in conjunction with an overall program of High-Tech health.

Why Does Brain Performance Decline?

There are many answers to that question. The brain suffers varying degrees of trauma throughout life that can impair its function, including aging itself. Head injuries, alcohol use, prescription and recreational drug use, free-radical accumulation, sugar consumption and glycation, the accumulation of pro-inflammatory compounds (AGEs), increased inflammatory damage of all kinds, poor circulation to the brain, high cholesterol, infections, and simple lack of stimulation can all cause damage to the brain's tissues. Both the brain's hardware (neurons) and software (neurotransmitters) can become damaged, resulting in faulty performance.

Other damage can be caused by the by-product of neuronal cell metabolism. This by-product is a kind of "cellular garbage" called *lipofuscion,* also called age pigment, which accumulates mainly in the brain and in the skin. When these accumulations become visible on your skin they're called liver spots. They are actually signs of tissue "spoilage," and as they build up in your brain, they inhibit and disrupt its normal activity, eventually causing the death of brain cells.

Excitotoxicity, damage caused by toxins in the brain, occurs when the brain loses control over the release of its own neurotransmitters, such as glutamate, serotonin, or dopamine. Like a leaky gas valve or malfunctioning meter, the brain then gives off inaccurate signals, resulting in imbalances between inhibitory and excitatory neurotransmitters, causing performance problems and destroying brain cells.

And then there's *cortisol,* the primary stress hormone, that is a major disrupter of the brain's efficiency because, as Dr. Barry Sears says in chapter 2, *"Nothing will kill brain cells faster than excess cortisol."*

So What's the Good News?

Despite all those possibilities for damage, there's plenty of good news! In the past, scientists thought that we lost brain cells as we age. Current research being conducted on the human brain, however, indicates that the brain keeps producing baby brain cells (stem cells) throughout its life. Some of this research is being conducted by Dr. Fred Gage of the Salk Institute in La Jolla, California. According to Dr. Gage, you don't find either a degeneration or a decline of cell volume in normal healthy brains; in fact, the number of neurons in the brain appears to remain constant as we age. What does occur is a loss of functional capacity. So the cells are there, even if they're not functioning as well as they used to (which wouldn't be true of Parkinson's or Alzheimer's disease, where you can see actual cell loss).

Scientists used to think that we lost brain function as we got older because we lost brain cells. According to Dr. Gage (and others), healthy brains do not lose cells, so whatever loss of function occurs comes from other sources.

In the future, the possibility for the replacement of lost or damaged brain cells, or the revitalization of senescent (aging) cells, may lie in the novel use of what are called *growth factors*. There are all sorts of growth factors in the human body, stimulating the development of everything from skin cells all the way up to—apparently—generating new neurons in old brains. A study conducted by Stem Cell Pharmaceuticals Inc. of Seattle, and reported in the *Proceedings of the National Academy of Sciences*, showed that introducing a cell growth factor called TGF-a into the forebrains of brain-altered rats stimulated brain stem cells to develop into healthy nerve cells that replaced damaged brain tissue. (This is a line of research unrelated to the poor results recently produced by implanting fetal stem cells into the brains of Parkinson's patients, which caused the disease to worsen.) The Seattle study was conducted using the rat's own brain stem cells, introducing the growth-inducing protein (TGF-a) to the stem cells already present and stimulating them to multiply and migrate to the injured sites (rather than transplanting cells from outside the brain). This procedure is on the current frontiers of neurological and medical research.

The Healthy High-Tech Power Brain Protocol

Suppose you want to begin to repair, maintain, and improve your cognitive efficiency right now. Do you have to wait until stem cells and growth factors can be implanted into your brain? Luckily, you do not. You can follow the protocols in the rest of this chapter to reach your own potential for maximum brain efficiency:

- **Since we know that the brain can continue to regenerate itself even into old age . . .**
  We now know how we can support this regenerative process.

- **Since we have been able to identify substantial risk factors that compromise the brain . . .**
  We now have many ways to counteract those risk factors.

The elements of achieving a Power Brain have been divided into two parts: **Preservation and Enhancement.**

Part 1, Preservation, lays out what you'll have to do to preserve the brain's structure and reduce cell damage. This is nuts-and-bolts maintenance, like flossing your teeth.

Part 2, Enhancement, contains information on "assisting" the brain's efficiency through the use of nootropics. It's important to note here that working with nootropics is like trying on a suit and seeing how it hangs. A suit that's perfect for me may not fit you well at all. That's what using a nootropic agent is like: you have to try it out and see if it fits. You may have to try on several "suits" before you find the one(s) that works best for you.

Part 1 of Achieving a Power Brain: Preservation

Here are seven important steps you can take to preserve (and begin to improve) your current state of brain efficiency:

Step 1: Implement the Paleotech Diet guidelines

Be sure to include plenty of fish and seafood. A diet high in fish oil has been shown to effectively reduce inflammation, which is a major cause of cell damage. Fish oil is a natural anti-inflammatory. Its consumption results in a somewhat different cell composition that produces less *arachidonic fatty acid.* If you consume more fish and seafood, your cells will contain less arachidonic fatty acid, which in turn means fewer pro-inflammatory eicosanoids (called cytokines) and other pro-inflammatory chemicals that can cause brain cell damage.

Epidemiological studies done worldwide (see chapter 2 on the Paleotech Diet) have amply demonstrated that frequent fish eaters enjoy much better overall health, including less cognitive impairment and lower incidence of Alzheimer's disease, than those who eat little or no fish. Since your brain is really made up of what you eat, there are obvious benefits in adding antioxidant-rich fruits and vegetables for preventing degenerative brain disorders.

Step 2: Cut down on sugar consumption

AGEs (again see chapter 2), which are the by-products of sugar consumption and are extremely harmful to brain tissue, may also be involved in the regulation of beta-amyloids—protein fragments that are one of the suspected causes of Alzheimer's disease, causing neuron destruction and generating the release of free radicals into the brain's tissues.

Step 3: Take an over-the-counter nonsteroidal anti-inflammatory

It turns out that inflammatory compounds in the blood are partially responsible for a whole host of common disorders, from atherosclerosis and colon cancer to Alzheimer's disease. The problem, when serious enough, can be defined as *chronic inflammatory syndrome*. The National Institute on Aging (NIA) has an ongoing study (forty years to date) called the Baltimore Longitudinal Study of Aging (BLSA). Researchers in the BLSA found a link between the use of anti-inflammatory drugs and a lowered risk for Alzheimer's disease. Men and women in the BLSA study who took NSAIDs (nonsteroidal anti-inflammatory drugs) regularly for as little as two years lowered their risk of developing Alzheimer's disease by as much as 60 percent.

Another NIA-supported study suggests that older people who regularly take aspirin or other anti-inflammatory drugs may be at lower risk of age-related cognitive decline (including Alzheimer's). A total of 7,671 older volunteers being studied as part of the Established Populations for Epidemiological Studies of the Elderly were monitored for changes in mental ability. Twenty-one percent were taking NSAIDs at the beginning of the study. At the end of three years, participants who used NSAIDs had *significantly* better cognitive function than those who hadn't taken them. On average, the volunteer taking NSAIDs had a cognitive ability equal to that of a person 3.5 years younger than their chronological age. NSAIDs reduced the risk of significant cognitive decline by about 20 percent.

NSAIDs currently on the market include the following:

- ibuprofen (Advil, Motrin)

- naproxen sodium (Aleve)

- indomethacin (Indocin)

- aspirin

- COX-2 inhibitors (Celebrex, Vioxx)

- plus newer versions likely to come on the market with reduced side effects

NSAIDs can have potential side effects, particularly stomach irritation and ulcers. Some people may have allergies or sensitivities to the ingredients. Always consult your physician about your plans to take NSAIDs, especially if you plan on taking them on a regular basis (and never take more than the recommended dosage).

A SIDE EFFECT—ADVANTAGE OR DISADVANTAGE?

There is one side effect of NSAIDs that may actually help brain efficiency. Prostaglandins are strong, hormonelike fatty acids in the body that can protect the stomach lining and promote blood clotting. NSAIDs inhibit prostaglandins. That's why they may upset your stomach. On the other hand, the fact that they work against blood clotting may actually work to your advantage, because they can decrease blood viscosity.

There are many factors that can affect blood viscosity, not all of them known (however, stress, excess cortisol, and immune-related inflammation are strong suspects). Dr. Steven Fowkes, founder of the Cognitive Enhancement Research Institute (CERI), explains that "the brain needs clear blood flow just like any other organ in the body, such as the liver or the heart. If the blood is too viscous, it's like trying to pour syrup out of a bottle that's just come out of the refrigerator. It takes its sweet time getting to your plate. On the other hand, if the syrup is less 'solid,' it will pour out freely.

"Your brain needs your blood (and the oxygen it carries) to flow freely. If your heart is pumping sludge, it's going to have a lot more work to do. Your heart will be stressed, plus your brain will be deprived of oxygen."

Here's an analogy: you travel the same highway to work every day. For years, the trip is fine. However, for many different reasons, the highway begins to be littered with broken-down cars. Now, your trip takes a lot longer because you have to drive around all these obstacles. Not only that, it now takes you sixty minutes to get to work instead of the twenty minutes it used to take. So by the time you get to work, you're already stressed out—and this pattern will only continue to worsen until you take steps to clear up the highway!

Step 4: Use neuroprotective antioxidants like lipoic acid

Since free radicals can do immense damage to brain cells, antioxidants are a necessary part of your Power Brain protocol. Glutathione (discussed in chapter 8) is a potent detoxifying amino acid and is highly protective of the brain. However, it is difficult to take orally, given its rapid breakdown by our digestive system. Fortunately, there are several antioxidants that convert into and/or raise levels of glutathione, chiefly **lipoic acid**, a vitaminlike proglutathione nutrient that is known to strengthen the entire antioxidant network. Lipoic acid is even more effective when taken along with vitamins C and E. (Note: Lipoic acid is also a potent anti-inflammatory; therefore, taking 10 to 100 milligrams per day may afford the brain double protection!)

Step 5: Reduce stress

The best way to fight stress is to avoid it as much as possible. Obviously, that is not always possible. Suffice it to say *again* that cortisol, your primary stress hormone, fries your brain cells, contributing to inflammation and all sorts of corollary damage to your brain and body. You can counter some of the ill effects of excess cortisol with a hormonelike nutrient called **pregnenolone**. Pregnenolone is also considered a smart drug that may be useful in memory enhancement, although that claim is not currently backed up by sufficient testing or documentation. According to Steven Fowkes, pregnenolone is a "plasticizing" nutrient, maintaining the brain's malleability and youthfulness.

Other important nutraceuticals for controlling stress damage are **magnesium** and **coenzyme Q_{10}** (CoQ_{10}). Magnesium is effective in controlling excess calcium damage to neurons; CoQ_{10} enhances the function of the mitochondria in our cells. (The mitochondria are the "energy factories" found inside of every cell, especially useful in the health of the human heart.)

Step 6: Exercise and enriched environments

According to an interview with Dr. Fred Gage, of the Salk Institute, in the August 2000 issue of *Life Extension* magazine, it is a known fact that new blood vessels form in the brain when we exercise. Apparently, the introduction of a new and enriched environment can also have the same effect.

Two separate studies were conducted on mice. One group was placed into a highly enriched environment that included many toys and other animals with whom they could interact. The results indicated that simply by enriching the environment, the total number of brain cells increased by 15 percent, a substantial amount relative to the size of the brain. Dr. Gage then conducted this experiment with older mice that had spent their entire lives in bare cages. The results show that neurogenesis (new neurons) coincided with increased performance of certain tasks for which they had been trained.

In the second experiment, mice were placed in a cage with free access to a running wheel for exercise. That group, too, showed an increase and proliferation in neurons. Both groups showed about double the amount of cells as the control group. Other studies have shown that old rats, when placed in enriched environments, solve mazes faster than rats in environments with no stimuli. In other words, it appears that these animals got "smarter" as a function of either stimulating their brains or exercising their bodies. The results of these experiments seem to indicate that stimulating the brain, through both environment and exercise, not only increases the number of brain cells but seems to improve cognitive function.

Scientists continue to study whether exercise alters the molecular mechanisms that are important for learning and memory. They're also weighing evidence that exercise prevents the negative effects of chronic stress on the brain and boosts the brain's capacity to ward off infection. These ongoing studies suggest that an active lifestyle—jogging, yoga, tai chi, and other specialized exercise regimens—not only maintains the function of the brain but may help repair damaged or aged brains. In their book *Aging and Cognition: Mental Processes, Self Awareness and Interventions*, Goggin and Stelmach maintain that physical exercise "can minimize and/or slow the rate of decline in some cognitive and physiological functions." In countless studies, physical exercise, which is routinely applied for the benefit of the cardiovascular system, has been demonstrated to be essential for the benefit of the brain and its performance.

It is now apparent that "novelty," the task of learning new things throughout your life, also helps to maintain or increase healthy brain performance. The "nun study," research being conducted with the School Sisters of Notre Dame through the University of Kentucky's Chandler Medical Center, has shown the ongoing and positive effects of *continued learning* throughout life. Researchers found significant evidence of the connection between longevity among the nuns and their levels of education. Cognitive function is sustained by active social involvement also; over thirty years ago the noted gerontologist Robert Butler found relationships between physical measures of cerebral physiology and social function. In his book *The Façade of Chronological Age* (University of Chicago Press, 1968), Butler wrote that maintenance of social contacts, social responsiveness, and goals in living were all associated with better brain function. The bottom line? Stay physically and socially active, and keep learning new stuff till the day you die. This may not sound exactly High Tech, but it may turn out to be extremely important in maintaining brain efficiency.

Step 7: Get sleep or get dull

If you now think exercise is important to your quality of life, get this: healthful sleep may turn out to be the single most important factor in predicting longevity, possibly more so than diet, exercise, or heredity. This is according to Dr. William Dement, author of *The Promise of Sleep*, and the world's leading authority on sleep, sleep deprivation, and the diagnosis and treatment of sleep disorders. It's impossible in this limited space to reproduce all his information indicating the central role of getting adequate sleep in the brain's capacity to learn, store information, and form long-term memories. According to Dement, a portion of sleep called REM (rapid eye movement) sleep may be a factor that helps memories "stick." Your productivity and performance will categorically suffer to the extent that you suffer sleep deprivation. The effects of fatigue obviously cause major disruption in brain function. It appears that personal sleep requirements are a fixed thing like body temperature, with very few people able to overcome this need. Sleep debt is a formula for disaster and for reducing the brain's efficiency in every measurable respect.

Part 2 of Achieving a Power Brain: Enhancement

There's much more to cover on the brain than can fit between the covers of this book, especially as we accelerate into the era of *genomic medicine and science* and try to make sense of the brain's intricacies and our notions of mind and subjectivity.

The brain performs in many ways to ensure our survival. It integrates, initiates, and controls functions in the whole body, with the assistance of sensory and motor nerves outside of the brain and the spinal cord. The brain is control central for thinking, cogitation, temperament, mood, character, personality, and our senses. Everything we do occurs as a result of complex chemical processes that take place in the brain. The brain regulates autonomic or automatic body functions (like digestion) that don't require our conscious participation. In addition to its billions of neurons, there are glial cells (up to fifty times the volume of neurons), which surround, support, and nourish neurons. Neurons communicate with each other and with sensory organs by producing and releasing neurotransmitters. These neurotransmitters carry messages between neurons in a complex molecular dance, involving docking sites called receptors, opening and closing nerve cell interiors, or kicking off other "dances" that determine what a receiving nerve cell will do. Some neurotransmitters inhibit cell function, making them less likely to act; others stimulate them to become active in some manner. Millions of signals go through the brain in fractions of seconds. Some neurons are involved in thinking, some in learning, others in remembering, planning, and even imagining.

The Formulas, Nutrients, and Nootropics

The brain depends on the healthy functioning of three dynamic mechanisms:

- communicating information

- using energy

- repairing cells and tissues

These dynamic elements can be vastly assisted by the use of many different nutrients, including ones that are now so commonly used they are almost considered mainstream, for instance:

Supplement	Amount per Day
Acetyl-L-carnitine	1,000 mg
Ginkgo biloba	500 mg
Choline	100 mg
St. John's wort	600 mg
Pregnenolone	20 mg
DMAE	250 mg

(See chapter 5 on nutraceuticals for a full listing of appropriate supplements.)

Moving into the High-Tech future, however, means moving into the world of smart drugs called *nootropics*. The main features of nootropic drugs are:

1 Under clinical conditions, they enhance learning. They also protect the brain from losing learned behaviors.

2 They facilitate the movement of information within and between the brain's hemispheres.

3 They strengthen the tissues of the brain and their resistance to physical and chemical injuries.

4 They increase the efficiency of the cortical and subcortical control mechanisms of the brain.

5 They have extremely low toxicity and few (if any) side effects.

These definitions of a nootropic drug were first proposed by C. E. Giurgea, the principal researcher and research coordinator for UCB, the Belgian company that launched the world's best-known, most studied, and arguably most effective nootropic drug ever, piracetam.

Piracetam This is the most popular smart drug for healthy, normal people. It is a broadly effective enhancer of human performance. Hundreds of studies have been done on its merits for normal healthy adults, normally aging individuals, and, beyond that, for people suffering from overt cognitive disorders. It is extraordinarily effective in reducing fatigue and improving your capacity to stay focused. Like other nootropics, it may postpone or even reverse "acceptable" brain aging. Technical information on piracetam and related nootropic agents is available in the groundbreaking books *Smart Drugs I & II* by Dr. Ward Dean and John Morgenthaler (Health Freedom Publications), *The Physician's Guide to Life Extension Drugs* from the Life Extension Foundation, and *Mind, Food and Smart Pills* by Ross Pelton (Doubleday). Using piracetam can improve individual learning potential and information retention, reaction time, mood, sensory perception, sexual arousal and response, energy levels, and memory.

Of all the "racetam" nootropics (there are also oxiracetam, pramiracetam, and aniracetam), piracetam is the one I have the greatest experience using and highest fondness for, in terms of its effect (it makes me feel wonderful) and its comfort. It greatly reduces fatigue. Not only is it well tolerated, safe, and virtually nontoxic, it has also been used to treat people who have had a concussion, are withdrawing from alcohol, or suffering from dyslexia and various forms of dementia. There is also documentation showing it protects the brain from prescription sedative overdose and electroconvulsive shock treatments (for the complete overview of research studies and broad applications of the "racetams," go on-line and read the article on nootropics by James South, M.A., "Nootropics—reviewing piracetam and analogues," at www.smart-drugs.net).

It is clear that sustained learning into the middle and older ages has become a matter and a requisite of staying competitive. If you want to stay in the game, marketplace realities demand that you keep up with people substantially younger than you in terms of productivity, tolerance for stress, and intellectual contribution. Piracetam is a potent tool in maintaining a competent edge: a typical dose range is 200 to 1,500 milligrams, spread throughout the day. Piracetam has a strong feel to it and may keep you up if taken late in the evening. Piracetam is not available in the United States, but it can easily be ordered from most overseas and Internet pharmacies. It comes in both injectable and tablet form.

Pyroglutamate (with arginine) This is an amino acid found naturally occurring in all foods, especially fruits and vegetables. It is closely related in structure to the "racetams," but has a weaker nootropic activity. (I call it "piracetam junior.") It is, however, available right at your local health food store, often in combination with *arginine*, another well-studied amino acid. In combination, this product improves the levels of *nitric oxide* in the body, a potent neurotransmitter associated with memory. Nitric oxide dilates blood vessels, improving blood flow to the brain. Pyroglutamate is known to improve memory and learning. And, if you are involved in intense physical activity or exercise, using pyroglutamate arginine will also assist in stimulating energetic processes of the brain, producing mild elevation, not unlike caffeine (without the side effects). It even supports the "natural" elevation of growth hormone levels within the body.

Vinpocetine Vinpocetine is an extract of periwinkle that has been shown to be a cerebral *metabolic* enhancer and a *selective cerebral vasodilator.* It has been shown to enhance oxygen and glucose uptake from the blood by brain neurons and to increase neuron ATP (energy molecule) production, even under low oxygen conditions (like high-altitude climbing). Vinpocetine is also an exceptional mood brightener. It is useful for anyone noticing a decrease in memory, alertness, or concentration, learning speed or learning ability. It also improves microcirculation to the eye by helping to unclog clumps of platelets that build up in the microvessels leading to the eyes and consequently to the brain. It has also been demonstrated to relieve headaches, including migraines. It effectively activates a group of neurons (called the *locus coeruleus* neurons) whose nerve fibers diffuse throughout the cerebral cortex, which improves all levels of cognitive function. This ability alone makes it a true "cognition enhancing agent." This product is effective either by itself or as part of a formulation, such as Memoractive by Thorne Research or Brain Wave Plus by Nutricology. Vincaclear by Life Enhancement is currently one of my favorite formulations, combining vinpocetine with arginine and vitamin C for better absorption. Vinpocetine helps correct many aspects of neuropathology having to do with conditions that compromise the brain's oxygen and energy requirements, such as strokes or cerebral arteriosclerosis.

Hydergine revisited This smart drug first hit the scene in a big way through the blockbusting bestseller *Life Extension,* by Dirk Pearson and Sandy Shaw, in the early eighties. Hydergine increases stores of the universal energy molecule ATP. It improves utilization of glucose in the brain and also enhances cerebral microcirculation. It is FDA-approved for "persons over sixty who manifest signs and symptoms of decline in mental capacity." *The Physicians' Desk Reference* defines this decline as impairment in mood, self-care, cognitive, and interpersonal skills. The *PDR* reports that by using a special rating scale (the SCAG), it statistically (though modestly) showed observable improvements in mental alertness, short-term memory, orientation, appetite, and other cognitive parameters, as well as helping to minimize confusion, dizziness, and fatigue, when hydergine was used over a twelve-week period. This was achieved using a modest dose of 3 milligrams, whereas numerous other studies indicate substantially better results at higher doses of 5 milligrams or more.

A number of these products are available only through overseas markets or through on-line providers who will procure them for you. Always consult with your doctor on their uses first. Keep in mind that traditional medical practice does not always encompass the use of smart drugs. If your doctor objects to their use, you may want to find a Functional Medicine practitioner to help you reach your Power Brain goals. For further information and product sources check out:

www.hfn-usa.com (Health Freedom Nutrition)
www.oz.lef.org (Life Extension Foundation)
www.nubrain-store.com
www.life-enhancement.com
www.ceri.com (Cognitive Enhancement Research Institute)
www.smart-drugs.net

Hydergine has another important function: *it slows down the deposit of lipofuscion in the brain!* Neurons in the brain have extensions called dendrites that reach out from their bodies, similar to the way in which tentacles extend from the body of an octopus. Dendrites facilitate communication throughout the nervous system and are necessary for memory and learning. New learning requires new dendrite growth. This growth is spurred on by nerve growth factor (NGF). It appears that hydergine may be able to stimulate new dendrite fibers in the same way that NGF does, although the mechanism is not yet well understood. In long-term studies it has been shown to normalize systolic blood pressure, reduce cholesterol, improve energy, reduce ringing in the ears, and relieve fatigue and visual disturbances.

Galantamine This is a phytonutrient that is an extract from the common snowdrop plant. It begins by blocking the action of a key brain enzyme involved in Alzheimer's disease, acetylcholinesterase (AchE).

Galantamine destroys AchE's ability to damage acetylcholine (ACh; see chapter 5 on nutraceuticals). Age-related memory impairments, or ARMIs, may also be caused by a decline in acetylcholine production. If there is a breakdown in its production, if it is broken down too rapidly, or if its release is inadequate, you have *cholinergic dysfunction*. When you preserve acetylcholine, you preserve memory. ACh is a neurotransmitter needed to shuttle messages in the form of electrochemical impulses within the brain. Galantamine binds to ACh receptors directly and stimulates neuronal function. It specifically binds to nicotinic receptors, which play a crucial role in memory and learning. Studies have also shown it to be useful as a sexual arouser, stabilizing erectile function and eliminating premature ejaculation.

The High-Tech Fight Against Alzheimer's

Here are some scary statistics: according to the Alzheimer's Association, about four million Americans have Alzheimer's disease, and fourteen million will have the disease by the middle of this century unless a cure or prevention is found. About one in ten Americans over age sixty-five has the disease, and nearly half of those over eighty-five have it.

The onset of Alzheimer's is one of the greatest fears associated with aging. Most of us would rather die than lose who we are and become dependent upon the kindness of others.

Our brains deteriorate with age, just as our bodies do. There is some degree of deterioration detectable at autopsy in almost every person over the age of sixty-five. For most of us, this deterioration leads to the annoyance of intermittent short-term memory loss and slow response times. When the deterioration is severe, we can become completely disabled, unable to function on our own.

Scientists do not yet know exactly what causes Alzheimer's disease, although there are several theories having to do with "sticky proteins," "stringy tangles," and an Alzheimer's susceptibility gene called ApoEe-4. Because we still don't know the cause, it has been difficult to find the cure. The good news is that Alzheimer's research began only two decades ago, and immense progress has been made in an extremely short period of time.

Here are some of the most recent advances in Alzheimer's research:

Drugs There are now more than sixty drugs, designed to prevent or slow the development of the disease, in various stages of research. Some of those drugs are NSAIDs and COX-2 inhibitors. One of the latest drugs to be developed is galantamine, which seems to reverse memory problems with a minimum of side effects. It works by raising the brain's level of acetylcholine, a neurotransmitter that helps nerve cells communicate with each other (see chapter 5 on nutraceuticals). It works best on people with mild to moderate cases of Alzheimer's; patients with the most advanced cases were not helped at all. Some studies have also shown that certain cholesterol-lowering drugs (statins) can decrease the occurrence of Alzheimer's.

Nerve growth factor (neurotrophic factor) Another area of research on Alzheimer's has focused on an essential brain chemical called nerve growth factor (I told you those growth factors were important!). No one knows exactly how the growth factor works, but we do know that it helps injured cells regenerate themselves. Recently, a group of researchers from the University of California at San Diego took skin cells from older monkeys, inserted a gene that makes human nerve growth factor, and then injected the modified cells into the brains of four monkeys. The modified cells then began to produce their own nerve growth factor and appeared to revive brain cells. In April 2001, the first such implant was conducted on a California woman. Doctors hope to delay cell death, and in the most ideal outcome, improve functioning of the remaining cells. The gene therapy is not expected to cure the disease, but to alleviate some symptoms, such as short-term memory loss. The procedure targets specific cells deep in the brain in what is called the cholinergic system. This area of the brain is important for supporting memory and cognitive function and degenerates significantly in people who have Alzheimer's.

Vaccine People who have Alzheimer's disease have deposits of plaque that form in the empty spaces between nerve cells. This plaque may be formed by the overproduction of an enzyme called beta amyloid. A vaccine, developed by the Elan Corporation, seems to significantly reduce existing plaque and prevent further plaque from developing. In a December 2000 *Wall Street Journal* article titled "Alzheimer's Vaccine Shows Promise in Test," Dale Schenk, vice president of discovery research at Elan, explained that the vaccine ". . . works by prompting the body to produce antibodies that stick to beta amyloid in the brain. Those antibodies act as a beacon for scavenging immune-system cells, which engulf and destroy the plaque." If research continues to be successful in this area, the vaccine might be given to elderly patients who are at high risk for developing Alzheimer's, but who do not yet show symptoms.

Nutrition According to the Alzheimer's Association, research presented at the World Alzheimer's Congress 2000, a high-fat diet during early and midadulthood may be associated with an increased risk of developing Alzheimer's, especially in people with a marker called the ApoEe-4 gene. Researchers found that people with the ApoEe-4 gene who also consumed the highest-fat diets had a sevenfold higher risk of developing Alzheimer's than those with the marker who ate lower-fat diets.

Exercise A study published in the *Proceedings of the National Academy of Sciences* (March 2001) indicates that a research team from the University Hospitals of Cleveland, in Ohio, found for the first time that an inactive lifestyle may contribute to an increased risk of dementia in old age. The results of their study showed that people with Alzheimer's had on average taken part in fewer types of recreational activities for less time and at a lesser intensity throughout their lives. These activities included swimming, gardening, roller skating, and football. The study compared 193 patients with Alzheimer's along with a control group of 358 healthy people of the same age; the individuals were all of comparable social and educational background. The healthy group were more likely to devote more hours per month to leisure pursuit and were more likely to favor intellectual or physical activity over passive ones such as watching television. The researchers concluded, in part, "that the diversity of activities and intensity of intellectual activity were reduced in patients with Alzheimer's compared with the control group. These findings may be because inactivity is a risk factor for the disease or because inactivity is a reflection of very early subclinical effects of the disease, or both."

As you must have gathered by now, a Power Brain is not something that is accomplished overnight. It is accomplished over a lifetime. Do not, however, worry about what you have or have not done before. The best time to start building a Power Brain—and a Healthy High-Tech Body, for that matter—is right now.

8 The Injectables

Injectable nutraceuticals, intravenous
glutathione, European cell treatments

If you want to have a Healthy High-Tech Body, you also have to have a Healthy High-Tech attitude. That means opening yourself up to new possibilities, new technologies, and new theories of treatment and prevention. You should always be cautious when it comes to matters of health; however, you should also know what options are available to you.

This chapter is about options (remember, Pillar 3 is not about the requirements for a Healthy High-Tech Body, but about the options you have for reaching your Healthy High-Tech goals). These are options you may not have heard about before either because they are not practiced widely in the United States or because they are illegal here (even though they have been used in Europe for many decades and are common medical practices in Germany, France, Switzerland, and Italy).

However, you will be hearing more and more about these types of treatments as the state of American medicine moves toward High-Tech health.

"The problem has been with both patients and doctors," says Dr. François de Borne, former director of Evian Spa and practitioner of rejuvenative medicine in France. "Both think in terms of illness, not wellness. If you're not sick, you don't go to a doctor. If you're a doctor, you don't treat a patient who is not sick. Universities do not train doctors for prevention; they train them to treat disease. And that's it."

Things are changing, however. In 1998, Drs. Miriam S. Wetzel, David M. Eisenberg, and Ted J. Kaptchuck conducted a survey of the 125 medical schools in the United States (reported in the *Journal of the American Medical Association*, September 2, 1998). Of the 117 colleges that responded, 64 percent offered elective courses in complementary or alternative therapies, or included these topics in regular courses.

Many doctors, dissatisfied with the kind of care they were trained to provide, are moving away from the more "traditional" disease-based model of medicine toward a High-Tech wellness model. Many of these doctors have moved into the fields of **Functional and Environmental Medicine.**

These medical specialties have emerged not only to treat people from a wellness-based model but also to address the problems of individuals with illnesses that do not respond to conventional medical treatment. Often these are chronic problems, non-specific complaints that can add up to a variety of debilitating symptoms, such as fatigue, lethargy, headaches, depression, anxiety, ringing in the ears, impaired concentration, eczema, allergies, irritable bowel, and many other problems.

Functional and Environmental practitioners look at a multitude of factors that are at play in the development of compromised health, such as:

- food hypersensitivities

- biochemical individuality

- inhalant allergies

- nutritional status

- hormone imbalances

- sleep disturbances

- weakened immunity

- toxic exposures

Environmental Medicine (the study of the effects of the environment on our health; more specifically, the impact of the toxins in the environment) especially focuses on individuals who have suffered from toxic exposures and may be suffering from *multiple chemical sensitivities*. A person who is chemically sensitive is often adversely affected by chemicals and industrial waste exposures that are fairly well tolerated by the general population. For the sensitive individual, these exposures can be debilitating and can lead to what is now called "environmental illness."

Environmental Medicine was pioneered by doctors like Dr. William Rea, a cardiothoracic surgeon at Dallas Environmental Health Center, and Walter Crinnion, N.D., associate professor at Bastyr University (Kenmore, Washington) and specialist in Environmental Medicine. There are now well over seven hundred doctors practicing Environmental Medicine, and thousands practicing Functional Medicine. The tests, tools, and protocols that have come out of these two areas are now spilling over into traditional medicine, especially when it comes to the realm of **injectables**.

Injectable Nutraceuticals

The term *injectables* refers to the system of delivery used to introduce vitamin and mineral nutrients into the body (as opposed to taking them orally). Injecting these nutrients amplifies and speeds up their effects on the body. For example, in a study reported in the October 2000 issue of *Archives of Pediatrics and Adolescent Medicine*, researchers administered a single dose of magnesium sulfate or a placebo to thirty children ages six to eighteen experiencing moderate to severe exacerbation of their asthma. Immediately following the infusion, the magnesium group had a *significantly* greater percentage of absolute improvements in three different categories, with the improvement being greater at 110 minutes. In addition, 50 percent of the children who received intravenous magnesium were discharged to their homes, versus none of those who received the placebo. Researchers concluded "children treated with 40mg/kg of intravenous magnesium sulphate for moderate to severe asthma showed remarkable improvement in short-term pulmonary function."

Once again, it is apparently the method of delivery that made the difference.

There are many nutraceuticals that can be injected, but there are three in particular that have been shown to produce promising High-Tech results in maintaining and enhancing efficiency, the byword of High-Tech health: the Myers Cocktail, injectable glutathione, and vitamin B_{12}.

The Myers Cocktail

The Myers Cocktail is named for a Maryland physician who used intravenous injections of nutrients to treat a wide array of health problems among his patients. More recently, Dr. Alan Gaby, president of the American Holistic Medical Association and patron saint of complementary medicine, has popularized the "cocktail." The original premise of the cocktail was to override a poorly functioning digestive system; you could simply go directly to the bloodstream. When nutrients are injected intravenously, digestion is bypassed.

The Myers Cocktail is often used when other treatments fail or fall short. I've personally seen the overwhelming success of these treatments in hundreds of cases through the offices of Drs. Richard Firshein, Ron Hoffman, Robert Atkins, Lionel Bisson, and Woodson Merill—and these are only the physicians that I know personally, here locally in New York City! There are hundreds more doctors like them around the country who now offer this potent mix of nutraceutical ingredients as an effective adjunct treatment for:

- fibromyalgia

- chronic fatigue

- chronic depression

- weak immune response

- asthma

- congestive heart disease

- chemical injury

- immunotoxicity

The Myers Cocktail is extremely effective for optimizing performance in many ways:

1 It can "boost" your immune system, especially if you're overtired, run down, or are in the middle of a stressful situation—circumstances that normally produce wear and tear on the immune system and often lead to illness.

2 It can ameliorate the damaging effects of stress.

3 It can shorten the duration of a flu or cold you already have.

4 It can reduce or eliminate the effects of jet lag (taken either before or after you travel).

5 It can help repair a worn-out energy system.

6 It can improve focus and clarity of mind.

7 Taken at the first sign of a migraine, it can provide great relief (something I've personally experienced).

8 It can speed recovery from surgery (if not contraindicated) and dental work.

9 It can lighten and brighten your mood.

There are very likely additional uses that have yet to be discovered. Many elderly people find a new resurgence of well-being and improvement in a number of areas where they are chronically weakened. Athletes who are treated with Myers Cocktails report a decrease in recovery time from strenuous activity and injuries.

The Ingredients of a Myers Cocktail The ingredients of Myers Cocktails are not set in stone. They are adjusted for each patient, according to his specific ailments and complaints. However, the most common ingredients include:

- B complex—1cc

- Vitamin C—1 to 10cc or more; usually 220 mg/cc or 500 mg/cc

- Magnesium—1 to 4cc, either 20 percent chloride or 50 percent sulfate (my preference)

- Dexpanthenol (B$_5$)—1 to 2cc

- Calcium—1 to 4cc (not recommended in cardiac problems or older patients)

Many doctors also include the following:

Glutathione: an antioxidant with important applications in a variety of problems, especially for those with challenging brain disorders (see page 212), from 300 to 2,000 milligrams.

Glycyrrhizin: an injectable extract of licorice, used as an oral supplement and injectable because:

- It's a powerful anti-inflammatory.

- It stimulates the immune system.

- It is antiviral, inhibiting Herpes simplex and Varicella zoster (which causes chicken pox and shingles) and providing rapid decrease in hepatitis (specifically hepatitis B, but it also has applications in hepatitis C, by potentiating the effects of interferon).

- It protects and promotes liver function.

- It helps stabilize adrenal function, guarding against energy depletion.

- It is a potent antiulcer agent.

- The controlled and well-monitored use of DGL, especially as an injectable, is *a powerful tool for reducing inflammatory damage to the body.* It is a central product with broad applications in Chinese medicine, and a popular version is manufactured in Japan and is known as SNMC.

Mineral or vitamin formulations: may include selenium, zinc, chromium, or folic acid.

Piracetam: a powerful cognitive enhancer and the "father" of smart drugs! This is strictly available overseas, under the name Nootropil. This product's safety and effectiveness were so impressive that a new category of pharmaceuticals was created called the *nootropics,* which became known as "smart drugs."

Nootropics is from the Greek meaning "acting on the mind." I've covered the nootropics (more on piracetam) in the section on the Power Brain. According to *The Physi-*

cian's Guide to Life Extension Drugs, piracetam has been shown to "synchronize the spheres of the brain by anchoring information in the brain more securely and creatively," while acting as a powerful antioxidant. Piracetam is truly pluripotent. Piracetam protects the brain *while* enhancing the efficiency of all higher brain functions associated with learning and memory. This compound is non-FDA-approved, despite its long-term track record of safe use in multiple clinical applications throughout Europe and its practically nonexistent toxicity. For personal experimental use, it is available in both an oral and an injectable delivery system. It makes a substantial contribution to the basic "cocktail."

Glutathione

Glutathione is a chemical antioxidant (an amino acid, to be precise) that is critical for detoxification. It is also considered by many to be one of the most powerful anti-aging nutrients ever discovered. Apparently, glutathione "picks up" any toxic substances that have found their way into your body and escorts them out. It is a tripeptide, that is, a small protein made from three amino acids: cysteine, glycine, and glutamic acid. You also need sulfur (contained in the cysteine) and selenium to make it. Fish oil may also help your body produce more glutathione.

As we age, most of us have declining glutathione levels. There is some controversy about the best way to raise glutathione levels in the body, though there is little controversy that raising the levels is a desirable thing. (This is because some of the glutathione you take in a supplement gets broken down into its amino acids by your digestive juices, which doesn't happen if you take it in injectable form.) You can supplement by taking glutathione directly, or cysteine (see n-acetyl-cysteine), or glutamine (which stimulates your liver to make more glutathione).

Glutathione has been investigated as a potential suppressant of the HIV virus, at least in the test tube, by researchers at Harvard, Stanford, and elsewhere. Many complementary medicine centers use it as an important part of treatment for patients with Crohn's disease and ulcerative colitis. Glutathione plays a critical role in defending the body against free-radical damage, helps prevent cataracts and other eye conditions, and, perhaps most important, it is a significant booster of the immune system.

However, recent studies have shown an even more promising use for glutathione in treating Parkinson's disease and several other brain-centered neurological disorders. In the last decade of the twentieth century, scientists discovered that Parkinson's patients suffer from a profound deficiency in glutathione. That has led many doctors, especially Dr. David Perlmutter, director of the Perlmutter Health Center in Naples, Florida, and author of *Brainrecovery.com*, to the treatment of Parkinson's using intravenous glutathione (there seems to be no response to oral glutathione therapy). In a 1996 study, conducted at the University of Sassari in Italy, researchers administered glutathione intravenously to nine patients with early Parkinson's disease for thirty days. As a result, all of the patients had an average 42 percent decline in disability. The effects lasted for two to four months after the study ended. There did not seem to be any side effects, unlike with the more traditional treatment of using the drug L-dopa, which can cause nausea, dizziness, and even liver damage.

According to Dr. Perlmutter, "While L-dopa therapy may help to temporarily reduce the symptoms of Parkinson's disease, many scientific reports are now appearing in the medical journals warning that L-dopa therapy may actually increase free radical production and thus speed up the progression of the illness, causing patients to worsen more quickly." Dr. Perlmutter and others are also exploring the uses of intravenous glutathione for treating other brain disorders, including ALS (Lou Gehrig's disease) and Alzheimer's.

In Europe, and especially in Italy, injectable glutathione is available in a form called Tationil (300 or 600 milligrams). It is used over there as (among other things) an antidote for alcohol poisoning and toxic overload of drugs (prescription and otherwise), and as a powerful antidepressant and mood enhancer.

Vitamin B$_{12}$ Injections

A popular injectable that has been used even by traditional doctors for many years is vitamin B$_{12}$. In fact, physicians now give more B$_{12}$ injections than almost any other vitamin supplement. Vitamin B$_{12}$ is found naturally in all foods of animal origin, including dairy, eggs, meat, fish, and poultry. That is why some vegetarians suffer from vitamin B$_{12}$ deficiency, although it takes many years for that to occur. Vitamin B$_{12}$ has been used by physicians as an adjunct treatment for several conditions, including asthma, chronic fatigue syndrome, depression, high homocysteine levels, and pernicious anemia.

Vitamin B$_{12}$ deficiency can cause fatigue, and the injectable is often used to treat patients, especially the elderly, who complain of tiredness. In 1973, a study reported in the *British Journal of Nutrition* indicated that individuals who have normal levels of vitamin B$_{12}$ have increased energy after injections of this vitamin. Since then, B$_{12}$ has been a popular injection for an energy boost, especially among athletes and bodybuilders. Although no real side effects have been reported from taking B$_{12}$ shots, there may be negative interactions with other drugs you may be taking. As always, make sure your healthcare practitioner knows about all medications you may be taking before starting you on a new treatment or protocol.

European Cell Shots

The History of Cell Shots: Theirs and Mine

You would think that a treatment considered to be High Tech would come from a new idea or a new technology. This is not the case with European cell therapy. In fact, the basic theory behind this treatment was stated best in the sixteenth century, by a physician named Paracelsus. He wrote, "Heart heals the heart, lung heals lung, spleen heals spleen; like cures like." Paracelsus (and others before him) believed that the best way to treat illness was to use living tissue to bolster ailing or aging tissue.

The modern-day use of this treatment began in 1931 when Swiss physician Paul Niehans discovered the beneficial effects of what was to become "live cell therapy." A colleague who had accidentally removed a patient's parathyroid glands during the course of thyroid surgery summoned Dr. Niehans. It appeared there was little chance of the woman's surviving the day without these glands. A successful transplant was the only chance the surgeon had of saving her. Niehans, who was skilled in transplanting organs and glands, was called in. In those days, it was the practice to transplant a steer's parathyroid (you heard it right) into the patient. When Niehans arrived, he realized that the woman would not survive the operation, so he sliced up the organ into thin pieces, mixed the pieces in a saline solution, loaded them into a hypodermic needle, and injected the mixture into the fatally ill woman.

Not only did the woman recover, she went on to live another thirty years, well into her nineties. That was when cell therapy was born. Since then nearly seventy thousand people have gone to La Prairie, Niehans's clinic in Switzerland, in pursuit of these revitalizing treatments. Cell therapy is used broadly throughout the world; its largest practitioner base is Germany, where it is routinely used by thousands of physicians. It is also practiced in France and Italy, and in England, where the Stephan Clinic has treated more than thirty thousand patients.

That's Niehans's story of cell therapy. Here's mine:

I'm a runner. I've been a runner for many years. In 1989, I was obsessed with running. I loved to run; I lived to run. Running was and is a way that I manage my health, my energy, my moods. However, in the late eighties I found that my running had caused a great deal of wear and tear—and pain—in my hips. I was determined to keep running, so I pursued whatever treatments I could find. I tried acupuncture. A little relief, not much. A doctor prescribed a combination of painkillers and anti-depressants, which made the pain go away and also kept me high and dysfunctional. Another doctor actually told me that I would be a good candidate for hip replacement in a few years. At age thirty-seven, this was not something I wanted to hear.

At the time, I was working for a holistic clinic and came across some information about these "cell" treatments that were only available in Europe and Mexico. I read that some of these treatments had proven very effective in chronic joint problems. I wasn't sure if I believed all the information I read, but I was desperate. I found a clinic in Mexico; I was extremely impressed by the doctor who ran it and the evidence he presented about the effectiveness of cell shots. So I decided to go for it, and he gave me three shots in each hip.

The next day I experienced some discomfort (more from the needles than anything else). By the end of the week, I was jogging up and down the beach completely pain free. Since then, I have traveled to Europe every few years to repeat the treatments and continue to run as well as I ever did.

How It Works

There are many kinds of cell therapy, including blood transfusions and bone marrow transplants. That is not the kind we are talking about here. European cell shots refer to the injection of cellular material from organs, fetuses, or embryos of animals to stimulate the healing and repair of human cell tissue and counteract the effects of aging.

When cell therapy was first put into use by Dr. Niehans, the animal cells were taken "live" directly from the animal to the operating room. However, that did not allow for enough time for the animal cells to be tested for disease and sterility. In the 1950s, these animal cells began to be freeze-dried (like coffee). This way, the cells could not only be tested but also could be preserved for later use.

Cell therapy works because the fetal cells taken from animals have no antigens (proteins that produce allergic or antibody reactions in humans). So they are not rejected by human cells. The injected cells then circulate throughout the body until they recognize and congregate at the human counterpart of the organ from which they are taken (liver to liver, kidney to kidney, and so on). When the animal cells reach their target, they stimulate the human organ to function with renewed efficiency.

There are a variety of treatments available today:

Cell type combinations These shots are used for anti-aging and revitalization effects. Four types of cells are combined—pituitary, liver, connective tissue, and reproductive glands (male or female)—plus a fifth type, depending on what the individual patient needs (for example, liver cells).

Whole embryo ultrafiltrate injections Also used for anti-aging, they are also intended to stimulate connective tissue and muscles. These injections contain material from all areas of the embryo, and therefore target the whole body rather than one specific organ.

Antibody injections Human cells are injected into an animal, whose immune systems then manufacture antibodies in response. The antibodies are harvested from the animal, purified, and injected into the patient. This treatment works much the same way as gamma globulin to boost immunity. This is an area that many scientists feel holds a promising future in treating autoimmune diseases like lupus and rheumatoid arthritis.

The science of cell therapy has evolved significantly since Niehans injected his early version of a live cell extract. He went on to use the various organs and glands, taken from sheep, refining the process along the way. Not only did he demonstrate the effectiveness of these cell implants to revitalize aging individuals, he demonstrated their effectiveness in treating severe immunological problems, as well as underdeveloped, diseased, and age-damaged organs. He found, as have many doctors since then, that cell therapy is extremely effective in restoring sexual vitality. Cell therapy has been used to treat virtually every age-related disorder in the book, including cardiovascular diseases, bone diseases, kidney diseases, and arteriosclerosis.

One product line that I consider extremely beneficial is Regeneresen. At the beginning of the 1950s, Dr. H. Dyckerhoff of Germany isolated RNA from fetal and juvenile animal tissue and introduced it, under the name of Regeneresen, into the treatment of diseases. Our bodies lose protein as we get older; Regeneresen is designed to replace those necessary proteins, using injections of RNA from various cattle organs and tissues, and from yeast. This therapy has been used to treat cardiovascular disease, immune dysfunction, sexual dysfunction, and age-related degenerative disorders. There are at least seventy-two different Regeneresen therapies, but the most popular and effective anti-aging therapy is RN-13. It comprises RNA from thirteen different bovine organs, including the liver, spleen, kidney, heart, and cerebral cortex.

Precautions and Side Effects

Before you get any type of cell treatment, a trained therapist will give you a physical examination to determine the appropriate treatment. You will be given a test injection to make sure that you don't have any allergic reactions. Treatment is not always appropriate. Although some treatments have been thought to help prevent cancer, people who already have cancer are not always good candidates, since these treatments can stimulate cell growth. Cell therapy is not recommended if you have kidney disease, liver failure, or acute infections. Some side effects, such as fatigue, have been known to occur for up to two weeks following the treatment. Occasionally the body's immune system will reject the injected cells, and high fever will follow. Fortunately, these side effects are not long lasting.

Unless you are looking to cure a specific disease, you will most likely have these treatments several times, over several years. "If you only have the treatment once," says Dr. de Borne, "it won't change your life. However, what you do feel is something like being 'cool.' You feel less anxious, more relaxed. You feel more energetic and revitalized. You suffer from fewer allergies, you don't get the flu. I urge my patients to have treatments at least once a year."

Cell therapy is practiced in many countries in Europe, including Switzerland, in the Bahamas, and in Mexico. *It is not legal in the United States.* There is little scientific documentation to back up the claims of these treatments, although thousands and thousands of people have claimed to have reaped their benefits. And don't forget that these treatments are not covered by medical insurance and often cost several thousand dollars.

You can get some live cell treatments in oral form over the Internet. They are about 50 percent as effective as injected live cells. The only oral cell products I recommend are NatCell frozen cellular extracts. They can be found on the Net at www.nutritiondynamics.com. There is, however, little quality control over most of these products sold on the Net; use precautions when ordering.

Obviously, the protocols in this chapter are to be done under strict supervision of a healthcare provider. You should be tested for allergies to any of the preservatives in any of these drugs or nutrients. High Tech does not mean high risk. None of the protocols in this chapter constitute any levels of high risk. Like anything, including exercise, there are slight risks involved. But if you take the proper precautions beforehand, such as discussing it with your primary care physician, you can determine if the risk potential is acceptable.

Injectable nutraceuticals and cell treatments are not cure-alls, nor are they the fountain of youth; however, used as part of a program for ongoing High-Tech health, they can be very effective.

9 Human Growth Hormone

The secret of youthful aging

Here's what we know at the moment: fruit flies, roundworms, and yeast live longer when genes are manipulated to effect certain growth hormone functions. Here's what else we know: some of the flies with manipulated genes lived up to 85 percent longer than usual. We also know that they were all born dwarfs.

We're just beginning to understand how and why we age, and what—if anything—we can do about it. But we're not there yet.

It should be apparent by now that the efficiency of a Healthy High-Tech Body is an amalgam. There are plenty of things to do in the pursuit of a long-lived and relatively well-functioning body till the day we give up our last breath. To have a total Healthy High-Tech Body, you have to work every angle of this book to some degree or another. Some things may be more appealing than others in terms of how far they take you out of your comfort zone; some may be just too strange or scary for you to try. Nonetheless, you should know what's going on in the world of High-Tech health and be able to make informed decisions about all your options.

That's where human growth hormone (hGH) replacement therapy comes in. It's a very hot, and controversial, topic in the field of anti-aging medicine. Human growth hormone may turn out to be a very useful component of regulating aging and restoring youthfulness. Most likely, it will be one piece of a much larger puzzle.

Some people would have you believe that using hGH *is* the solution, the salient chemical addition that would make you a young vital stud or studdess again. It is probably not for everyone. With proper testing and supervision, however, *it could be the way to go, it could be the right fit for you.*

Human growth hormone is a substance that is produced naturally within the body, secreted by the pituitary gland to promote growth during adolescence. The production of hGH tapers off as we get older. HGH has been around for many years as a treatment for individuals (especially children) who are deficient in it, and who suffer from serious development problems in achieving proper height, muscle, and bone growth.

Currently it has achieved star status in anti-aging treatments because of its literal ability to reverse many of the apparent signs of aging, especially loss of lean muscle mass. HGH levels decline with age, and so does everything else that they touch on their way down. But when hGH is used safely, in proper dosing, both lean muscle mass and bone density increase, and body fat drops.

HGH replacement therapy came to my attention in 1996, as it did for many others, when a study reported in the *Annals of Internal Medicine* titled "Growth Hormone Replacement in Healthy Older Men Improves Body Composition but Not Functional Ability" appeared. The study was conducted by a blue ribbon panel of medical experts and researchers out of the University of California, the Department of Veteran Affairs Medical Center, and San Francisco General Hospital. The study concluded that "physiologic doses of growth hormone given for 6 months to healthy older men with well-preserved functional abilities increased lean muscle mass and decreased fat mass. Although body composition improved with growth hormone use, functional ability did not improve. Side effects occurred frequently."

So the study found that hGH did not affect participants' brain performance or cognitive efficiency. It found that there were frequent side effects. But it also found that the hGH had a definite positive effect. The fifty-two participants in the study ranged from seventy to eighty-five years old. They were healthy older men with well-preserved functional ability but with low levels of insulinlike growth factor 1 (commonly called IGF-1, an indicator of hGH levels in the body). After six months of treatments with hGH, the study showed that lean muscle mass had increased by 4.3 percent and that body fat had decreased by 13.1 percent in the growth hormone group compared with the placebo group. In a separate, unblinded trial quoted in this study, treatment in a group of men over sixty had increased lean muscle mass by 9 percent and decreased fat mass by 15 percent. There appeared to be some modest increase in muscle strength as well.

Other studies have linked the decline of growth hormone with many of the other symptoms of aging, including cardiovascular disease, wrinkling, decreased energy and decreased sexual function, osteoporosis, and more.

What Is Human Growth Hormone?

In a nutshell, hGH is one of many hormones that our bodies produce, including testosterone, estrogen, melatonin, and DHEA. It is the master hormone, if you will, the orchestra conductor for all factors that involve physical development. Children who suffer the effects of hGH deficiency are short in stature with small hands, feet, and skulls. Their teeth come in late, and their skin is thin and pale. Their nails don't grow well, and their voices may be high-pitched. Many of these children develop the fat around the middle that is also characteristic of hGH deficiency in adults. In addition, their bones are porous and their lean tissue mass is reduced; in hGH-deficient adults, the skin is thin and "crow's-feet" wrinkling is pronounced (people who have their pituitary gland

SOME CHARACTERISTICS OF GROWTH HORMONE DEFICIENCY

Anabolic tone

- reduced lean body mass/skeletal mass
- reduced exercise performance
- increased total body fat
- increased abdominal and visceral fat

Lipid effects

- elevated LDL cholesterol
- decreased HDL cholesterol
- elevated apolipoprotein-B

Bone effects

- lack of bone

Metabolic effects

- insulin resistance (in obese people)
- hypoglycemia
- possible abnormal resting metabolic rate
- reduced t4 to t3 conversion (thyroid hormones)

Protein synthesis

- thin skin
- lack of collagen
- decreased size of all organs
- decreased nail and hair growth

Dehydration

- reduced sweating/inability to thermoregulate
- reduced cardiac output (potentially)
- increased vascular resistance

Mental health

- reduced energy
- emotional instability
- depression
- poor memory and concentration
- reduced sex drive

(The above is adapted from *Growth Hormone in Adults: Physiological and Clinical Aspects*. Juul Anders and Jens Jorgensen [eds]. NY: Cambridge University Press, 1966.)

removed develop pronounced crow's feet). Some research has shown that hGH treatment increases serum type III procollagen, an important building block for skin and connective tissue. Decreased skin thickness and resultant wrinkles are signs of old age; increased skin thickness and smoother skin are evidence of successful hGH treatment.

Chemical messengers sent over from another part of the brain called the hypothalamus release growth hormone from the pituitary gland. It is released in four main bursts or "pulses" in young men and more often in young women. Most of this release occurs at night, in the beginning phases of sleep. If you read chapter 4 on fat burning, you know that in order to lose weight properly, you have to get adequate sleep, for this very reason. When you don't get enough sleep, you don't "pulse" hGH, and you lose its effects on regulating your fat deposition. HGH may be released about twelve times in a twenty-four-hour period, in small spurts throughout the day, determined by exercise and the foods that you eat.

Starting at about age fifty, the number and intensity of pulses decrease, at the rate of about 14 percent every decade, into old age to the point where some elderly people don't release any at all. A sixty-year-old individual might be secreting 25 percent of the hGH produced by a twenty-year-old; this decline is called *somatopause*. Just like menopause, where you have declining levels of estrogen and progesterone, and andropause, where you have declining levels of testosterone, there is somatopause, the drop in levels of growth hormones. But like in menopause and andropause, just because the levels go low doesn't mean that you necessarily need to do anything about it.

Currently hGH therapy is FDA-approved for adults with hGH deficiency. You can get a blood test to confirm your levels. The approval of a synthetic hGH called Humatrope, manufactured by Eli Lilly, is based on clinical data demonstrating its effectiveness in increasing lean muscle mass, decreasing body fat, increasing exercise capacity, and raising HDL ("good") cholesterol levels. Additional studies published in the *New England Journal of Medicine* and others show that hGH may reverse biological aging parameters by: restoring muscle mass, decreasing body fat, reducing wrinkling, restoring hair loss, increasing energy, increasing sexual function, improving cholesterol profiles, improving vision, normalizing blood pressure, improving immune function, and assisting in wound healing.

Life Extension Institute Study on Human Growth Hormone

One of the largest studies of the effects of hGH on humans took place at the Palm Springs Life Extension Institute, by Dr. Edmund Chien, institute director, and his associate, Dr. Leon Terry, a neuroendrocrinologist from the Department of Neurology at the Medical College of Wisconsin. The study, which has been widely cited, demonstrated that the use of low-dose, high-frequency hGH injections, in combination with other hormones, proved to be universally effective in *positively* improving the health of 202 patients. Here are the results of the assessment, entitled appropriately enough:

Assessment

Effects of Growth Hormone Administration

(Low-Dose Frequency) in 202 patients

L. CASS TERRY, M.D., Ph.D., and EDMUND CHIEN, M.D.

Medical College of Wisconsin and Palm Springs Life Extension Institute

STRENGTH, EXERCISE, AND BODY FAT	IMPROVEMENT
Muscle strength	88%
Muscle size	81%
Body fat loss	72%
Exercise tolerance	81%
Exercise endurance	83%
Skin and hair	
Skin texture	71%
Skin thickness	68%
Skin elasticity	71%
Wrinkle disappearance	51%
New hair growth	38%

Healing, flexibility, and resistance

Healing of old injuries	55%
Healing of other injuries	61%
Healing capacity	71%
Back flexibility	53%
Resistance to common illnesses	73%

Sexual function

Sexual potency/frequency	75%
Duration of penile erection	62%
Frequency of nighttime urination	57%
Hot flashes	58%
Menstrual cycle regulation	39%

Energy, emotions, and memory

Energy level	84%
Emotional stability	67%
Attitude toward life	78%
Memory	62%

These improvements occurred within one to three months of the onset of treatment, with a tendency to continue improving over six months of treatment. Drs. Chien and Terry believe in a comprehensive approach to deterring the aging process by monitoring hormone levels, along with exercise, diet, and stress reduction.

If You're Thinking About Using hGH

The use of hGH has become increasingly popular, especially for athletes and body-builders. It stimulates growth in all tissues, including muscle tissue, and may strengthen connective tissue, cartilage, and tendons. So besides making you look good and improving strength, it may reduce susceptibility to injury.

The use of human growth hormone can have its downsides. There have been one or two studies that seem to point to an association between higher levels of hGH and higher risk of prostate cancer. Other studies have shown no risk increase. Some people experience water retention and bloating (which can often be relieved by changing the dosage). In extreme cases, an excess of growth hormone can cause a disease called acromegaly, where the bones in the hands, face, and feet grow out of proportion to the rest of the body.

HGH must be prescribed by a doctor, and it should be monitored closely. It can only be administered by injection, because if swallowed, the hormone would not be absorbed by the body, it would be digested by it. That means you have to be willing to give yourself injections six days a week. And it is not cheap. The hGH alone costs about $600 a month, and then you still have to pay for the doctor or clinic fees. One of the leading clinical operations in this country using hGH replacement therapy bundled in with additional "anti-aging treatments" is a clinic in Las Vegas, Nevada, called Cenegenics.

The Cenegenics Experience

Cenegenics is one of the highest-profile anti-aging clinics in the United States. This is a clinic with muscle. It is extremely upscale. Since the program tends to be expensive, the clients tend to be wealthy. Most are looking for ways to stay young. It is not at all out of place in Las Vegas.

Since I wanted to learn more about hGH and anti-aging clinics in general, I decided to find out for myself. What I found was a clinic with a top-flight staff of doctors, researchers, exercise physiologists, nutritionists, and extensive support personnel. Before anyone even mentions hGH replacement therapy, they do state-of-the-art diagnostic testing, top to bottom. At the base of their testing is the MEDBACE (Medical Biological Age Comprehensive Evaluation) test. This involves testing twelve different biomarkers of aging, memory, cognition, lung function/capacity, vision, hearing, muscle motor tests, and so on. They do body fat measurements, skin thickness and elasticity, and bone mineral density. Two weeks before you arrive at Cenegenics, a blood sample is taken at your home (they arrange for a local phlebotomist to come to your home and draw the sample). They take a complete medical history. The point of all this is not only to find out your current health status but also to determine your "real age," as opposed to your chronological age.

Cenegenics is a proponent of hGH therapy—but only in conjunction with a total health program.

"The most obvious effect of hGH is that it increases quality of life," says Dr. David Leonardi, medical director of Cenegenics. "But we have to realize that these hormones are a double-edged sword. It's not enough to just look at the low level of a hormone and supplement it to raise the level. It's going to affect several other parameters in the patient's chemistry and possibly affect other hormone levels as well. That could be detrimental. So you have to look at what that particular patient's chemistry shows and what they may be at risk for. It's not just a simple issue of supplementing a hormone, because there's a cascading effect that takes place. That's why patients have to be closely monitored."

For example, Dr. Leonardi points out the fact that hGH can help a patient burn more fat. With hGH treatments, prefatty acids are delivered from the fat cells to the blood cells and can then be picked up by the muscle cells and burned for fuel instead of glucose. So you become slightly more insulin resistant. "That's a wonderful thing if you're on a low glycemic diet," says Dr. Leonardi, "because you get the best of both worlds: you burn fat and your muscle cells get fuel, and insulin resistance becomes a non-issue." So if you're on a low glycemic diet and you take growth hormone, your blood sugar levels will actually drop over time.

But what if you're a couch potato and you eat junk food—and then you take hGH? Because of the insulin resistance that you're developing, your blood sugar levels will gradually increase. Which brings us back to the amalgam of the Healthy High-Tech Body. You cannot take hGH and expect that it will solve all your aging problems. It, like all other aspects of the Healthy High-Tech Body, must be combined with a proper diet and exercise.

Cenegenics will monitor your progress through ongoing blood testing when you get back home. It should be emphasized that Cenegenics practices Prevention with a capital P. So although they specialize in the application of hGH replacement therapy, they practice a combination of optimal protocol, intense patient management, highly refined service, and comprehensive diagnostics. This is among the better preventative medical operations you'll find in this country, should you decide to use hGH replacement therapy.

Growth Hormones and Regenerative Medicine

Human growth hormone is being studied for many specific uses, all part of what is being called **regenerative medicine**—the science of stimulating cells to regenerate themselves and/or stimulate other cells to regenerate. When this aspect of our medical future arrives, it will make hGH therapy look positively primitive. For instance, one study recently injected a growth-producing protein called TGF-a into the brains of rats that had a Parkinson's-like disease. The protein stimulated brain cells to develop into nerve cells that replaced damaged brain tissue. Human growth hormone, combined with a high protein diet, has been shown to ease the symptoms of Crohn's disease. Crohn's disease causes abdominal pain, bleeding, and a breakdown of the intestinal wall. One study theorized that the hGH helped rebuild damaged tissue in the intestinal wall.

There is another growth factor, known as *keratinocyte growth factor*, or KGF2, currently in trials to test its effectiveness. KGF2 is a protein that stimulates the cells of the skin and inner body linings to heal wounds and is being tested on people with ulcers that don't heal. As scientists identify other similar growth factors, regenerating a whole new outer (that is, youthful) skin may become common.

Then there is the amazing Dr. Dunn. While channel surfing during a vacation in Florida, I came across a news segment on an orthopedic surgeon named Allan Dunn who was doing something remarkable. He was injecting hGH directly into injured joints; some fractured, others damaged by the wear and tear of use. His results are amazing: his patients are experiencing actual repair of their damaged joints. Using a number of research tools, including fluorescent antibody markers, Dr. Dunn discovered that cartilage, which is the tissue found within joints, has at its surface a specialized microvascular system, consisting of tiny blood vessels, that had previously been undiscovered. This discovery led Dr. Dunn to the development of intra articular growth hormone (IAHG). Dr. Dunn observed that in adults with acromegaly, the excess hGH they produced would cause the overexpansion of cartilage. He reasoned that if hGH had this effect on cartilage, maybe it could be directly injected into joints to promote the growth of new cartilage that had deteriorated. Eventually, he was able to show that injecting growth hormone into the joints of research animals would restimulate the growth of the microvascular system (which he named the glomeruloids). It appears that IAGH telegraphs to the body the required signals to generate new cartilage, creating conditions not unlike those that exist in the body of a child, growing and making new joint tissue. Dr. Dunn believes that as a first-line therapy this may be an effective step to take to restore healthy cartilage and joint function (for more information on contacting Dr. Dunn, see the resource guide).

And, getting back to the old but tiny fruit flies mentioned at the beginning of this chapter, many scientists believe that growth hormones are the key to extending the human life span. Give them a few more years to work out the kinks, and they will figure out how to add at least forty healthy years to our lives.

10 Diagnostics

The new paradigm in medicine

There is no way of knowing, at this pivotal point in discovery and exploration, exactly where medicine is heading. Every *Star Trek* fan has seen that in an imagined future, physicians will be able to run a handheld device over your body, diagnose your problem within seconds, and heal your illnesses and injuries within minutes. We are still a long way from that reality (We're doctors, Jim, not magicians!); however, we are getting closer to it every year.

One of the reasons is the paradigm shift that is slowly taking hold of medicine. It has taken us centuries to figure out just how the body works; we're just beginning to understand how to fix it when it gets into trouble. We don't know all the answers yet, of course, but we have made great progress.

Now, however, many medical practitioners are saying, "We don't want to wait until patients get sick and then try to help them. We want to help them avoid getting sick in the first place." That's how Functional Medicine was born (see chapter 8).

In the twentieth century, scientists began to study not only how the body works but how disease works as well. They looked at patients with heart disease, for instance, to discover what they all had in common. One of those discoveries was that many people with heart disease had high levels of LDL or "bad" cholesterol. Further study revealed that lowering LDL cholesterol levels reduced heart attacks in men and women by one-third. As a result, people now get regularly tested for cholesterol levels so that they can take action *before* their LDL gets them into serious medical trouble.

Elevated LDL levels became known as a "marker," or predictor, of heart disease. Every day, new markers, or predictors, are being discovered for all kinds of diseases: heart disease, cancer, digestive disorders, hormonal imbalances, brain performance. Every day, new ways of testing for these markers are also being discovered, some as simple as a blood test or urine sample, and others highly complex technical advancements.

Some of these tests are standard medical practice. Some are outside the norm of traditional medicine. Some have been embraced by physicians everywhere; some are still highly controversial. And because most doctors are still steeped in the "treat the disease" mode of healthcare, it will likely be up to you to bring up the subject of many of these tests.

A large part of High-Tech health is knowing where you are, healthwise, at any given point in time. Given that the underlying theme of High-Tech health is maximizing your body's efficiency, you need to determine your current states of efficiency within the body's various systems. You want to be able to measure your health as precisely as possible, and then take whatever steps are necessary to build, preserve, or repair efficiently. So if you want to develop and maintain a Healthy High-Tech Body, you need to know about the diagnostic procedures in this chapter—and discuss them with your doctor and/or health professional.

This chapter will cover four important areas of diagnostic testing you should know about:

1. The basics These are the baseline tests, most of them approved by even the most traditional of doctors, to determine how healthy you are in a variety of areas. These tests become more important as you age and are the foundation of High-Tech health.

2. Heart disease markers This is one of the fastest-growing areas of medical science. It seems that there are many new ways of predicting heart disease, and we should be checking for all of them.

3. Functional assessments These tests come from the field of Functional Medicine and are designed to evaluate your current state of health (as opposed to your current illness) so that you can take any appropriate preventative measures and make lifestyle, supplemental, and nutritional adjustments before disease occurs.

4. High-Tech scanning These are the latest advancements in technology-based diagnostic tools.

Diagnostic Testing Part I

The Basics

These are tests that may not be particularly High Tech in and of themselves but are essential to High-Tech health. Even if you've had a physical and passed with flying colors, remember that many doctors are pressed for time—and many of them are feeling the financial squeeze from HMOs. So they may inadvertently be skimping on tests you should have, especially if you are over forty.

Here are the fundamental tests you should not do without:

If you are under forty (these are for factors that lower efficiency at any age, depending on genetics and lifestyle):

Cholesterol A simple blood test can tell you if you have elevated LDL. Your total cholesterol level should be less than 200, your LDL level less than 130, and your HDL ("good") level above 70.

Blood pressure Although blood pressure increases with age, young people as well as the elderly can suffer from high blood pressure. And if you let it go, it can cause serious damage. If you have high blood pressure, it indicates that there is excessive force being used by the heart to pump blood throughout the body, which means it has to work harder than it should to get blood and oxygen to the body's organs and tissues. Over an extended period of time, this tends to enlarge and weaken the heart. Arteries become hardened and lose elasticity. All of this can lead to heart attack, stroke, kidney failure, and atherosclerosis.

WARNING There are *no symptoms* for high blood pressure—which makes this test incredibly important! You should have it checked every time you see your doctor, and there are now many kits you can buy to check your pressure at home.

Some factors that increase the likelihood of high blood pressure are race (African Americans are particularly prone), age, obesity, smoking, and sedentary lifestyle. There are also many medications (prescription and over-the-counter) and supplements that tend to increase blood pressure, so always let your doctor know what you are taking. Optimal blood pressure levels are 120/80.

Pap smear All women over the age of eighteen should have an annual Pap smear. The newest development in this area is the **thin prep Pap smear**. The test is the same as a regular Pap smear, except that instead of smearing cervical cells onto a slide, the doctor rinses the cells into a vial and sends it to a lab that filters out blood and mucus, which can potentially obscure cancerous cells. Some studies have shown this test to be 65 percent more effective in detecting abnormalities than traditional Pap smears.

If you are in your forties, add:

Mammograms After the age of forty, women should have mammograms every one to two years. If you have particularly dense breasts, which are more difficult to read by mammogram alone (ask your doctor about this), you might want to ask for a mammogram plus ultrasound. The ultrasound is a noninvasive procedure that uses sound waves to view the breast.

Skin cancer screening test   There are about fifty thousand new cases of melanoma each year in the United States, and almost eight thousand of them will die from this disease. See a dermatologist once a year for a skin checkup, especially if you have spent a lot of time in the sun, have a family history of melanoma, have more than ten moles, or have moles that are irregularly shaped or strange in color.

If you are in your fifties, sixties, and seventies, add:

Prostate exam   There are several methods of testing for prostate cancer. First, there is the basic digital rectal exam performed by a urologist to determine if you have an enlarged prostate. Then there is the PSA test. PSA stands for prostate specific antigen, a protein produced by both benign and malignant prostate cells. The normal range of PSA level is between 0 and 4. A PSA of over 10 is a strong indication of cancer. The American Cancer Society recommends that men fifty and over get screened for prostate cancer once a year.

> **NOTE**   If you are taking any supplements (like saw palmetto) for prostate health, it is important to let your doctor know. Some urologists recommend that you get a baseline PSA level before you begin taking such supplements and then continue with your yearly checkups.

Colorectal cancer screening

Colorectal cancer is the second-leading cause of cancer death in the United States. If detected early, it has a good cure rate. There are several screening methods for this disease:

- **Fecal occult blood test (FOBT):** a stool test that looks for microscopic amounts of fecal blood. This test is only 30 percent effective in detecting early cancer and should be performed once a year in conjunction with the other screening methods.

- **Flexible sigmoidoscopy:** an endoscope—a flexible tube with a light and a camera on the end—is inserted into the rectum and lower third of the colon. This test checks for polyps, benign growths that can turn cancerous, and should be performed every five years.

- **Colonoscopy:** similar to the sigmoidoscopy, except that it examines the entire colon. This process is done under sedation and should be performed every ten years (more often if you have high-risk factors such as a family history of colorectal cancer or a personal history of colitis or Crohn's disease).

Bone mineral density (BMD) testing This test, which determines the density of your bones, screens for osteoporosis. It uses sound waves or small amounts of radiation, and your results are compared with the average BMD of a healthy young adult. A BMD test can detect bone loss at an early stage; normal X rays are not strong enough to detect bone loss until at least 30 percent of bone mass has been lost. Women who have been receiving hormone replacement therapy for a prolonged period are urged to have this test done. Although it is more common in women, men can suffer from osteoporosis too, so you should consult your doctor about the necessity for this test. BMD testing usually takes about five minutes, you don't need to undress for it, and there is no special preparation necessary.

Diagnostic Testing Part II

Matters of the Heart: Twenty-First-Century Markers

We all know the major risk factors for heart disease—abnormal cholesterol levels, obesity, smoking, family history, diabetes, lack of exercise. In the last few years of the twentieth century, however, scientists began to make a worrisome observation:

some patients with no apparent risk factors were turning up with serious heart disease. Therefore, there had to be other, heretofore unknown risk factors that could lead to the disease.

As the twentieth century gave way to the twenty-first, more and more of these markers were discovered (and there will probably be even more as time goes by) in four main areas:

- nutritional deficiencies: homocysteine and iron

- inflammation and infection: C-reactive protein

- blood clotters: fibrinogen

- genetically determined factors: lipoprotein (a)

These new risk factors are cumulative; the more you have, the greater your chances for developing heart disease. The good news is that most can be detected by simple blood tests and controlled by following the Paleotech Diet guidelines and adding appropriate supplements. Research is continuing as to the origins of these markers and the solutions to their presence.

Here are four of the most important twenty-first-century markers:

Homocysteine   The dangers of high levels of homocysteine are discussed in chapter 5 on nutraceuticals. However, just to reinforce that message, elevated levels of homocysteine have been linked to increased risk of premature coronary artery disease, stroke, and blood clots. A recent study reported in *Arteriosclerosis, Thrombosis, and Vascular Biology* found that there was a linear relationship between blood homocysteine levels and the severity of coronary blockages: For every 10 percent elevation of homocysteine, there was nearly the same rise in the risk of developing severe coronary heart disease. High homocysteine levels can be controlled by taking B_6, B_{12}, and folic acid.

Iron We all know that it's important to get enough iron. However, some studies now show that too much iron in the blood can contribute to heart disease. In his book *Heart Sense for Women,* Dr. Stephen Sinatra states that "no one is yet sure exactly how elevated levels of iron contribute to heart disease, but researchers have a number of ideas. Some research has indicated that iron . . . may play a role in causing the formation of free radicals, which oxidize LDL cholesterol in the blood, making it more likely to adhere to artery walls to form plaque."

C-reactive protein (CRP) This protein is a sensitive marker of inflammation and is released into the bloodstream any time there is active inflammation in the body (due to infection, injury, or various conditions, such as arthritis). A 1998 study measured C-reactive protein levels obtained from 39,876 healthy, postmenopausal American women. The study showed that the women who had the highest levels of C-reactive protein had a fivefold increase in the risk of developing cardiovascular disease, and a sevenfold increase in the risk of having a heart attack or stroke. As of now, there is no clear treatment for elevated levels of CRP. Since CRP is a marker of inflammation, usually caused by some kind of infection, it is thought that antibiotics may be an effective treatment. There are also studies under way to determine whether *statin* drugs, used to treat high cholesterol, may be useful in lowering CRP levels.

Fibrinogen This is a blood-clotting factor, which can cause hypercoagulation and excessive blood thickening. Both fibrinogen and C-reactive protein are produced in the liver by pro-inflammatory cytokines (a group of protein compounds that can cause tumors and cancer). Studies have shown several facts about fibrinogen: (1) people with high levels of fibrinogen were twice as likely to die of a heart attack; (2) smoking can greatly contribute to high fibrinogen levels; and (3) fibrinogen levels go up as estrogen goes down. Therefore, estrogen replacement therapy can significantly reduce fibrinogen levels. High doses of fish oil, olive oil, vitamin A, and vitamin C have also been shown to reduce fibrinogen levels.

Lipoprotein-associated phospholipase [Lp(a)] This is another marker that indicates the likelihood of inflammation of the heart and arteries. Lp(a) flows through the blood with LDL and is one of the components that makes LDL "bad." Unfortunately, however, lowering your LDL level does not always lower your level of Lp(a). High Lp(a) is largely an inherited factor. Like fibrinogen, Lp(a) levels tend to increase as estrogen decreases. Some supplements that have been shown to lower Lp(a) levels include coenzyme Q_{10}, vitamin C, and niacin.

Triglycerides New research has demonstrated that elevated triglyceride levels put you at the highest risk of all for heart attack. Triglycerides are fats composed of three (*tri*) fatty acids attached to a sugar-based (*glycerol*) molecular backbone. Triglycerides are used as fuel throughout the cells of the body. Most of your stored body fat, especially around your gut and middle, is stored triglyceride. High triglycerides means increased insulin resistance. When both insulin and triglycerides rise, the risk for heart disease rises right along with them.

Testing Your Blood for Heart Disease

The bad news is that most traditional doctors will not offer these tests as part of routine examinations, and insurance may not cover your costs. The good news is that many doctors will perform these tests if you ask for them, and they are not usually very expensive.

The January 2001 issue of *Life Extension* magazine published the following chart, which includes what they call the "standard reference range," or what doctors will tell you is a normal range for the markers discussed above, and the "optimal" level, which is what the Life Extension Foundation considers to be the level you want to maintain:

Blood test	What the "standard reference range" allows	The "optimal" level you want to maintain
Cholesterol	Up to 199 mg/dL	Between 180 and 220 mg/dL
LDL cholesterol	Up to 129 mg/dL	Under 100 mg/dL
HDL cholesterol	No lower than 35 mg/dL	Over 50 mg/dL
Homocysteine	Up to 15 micro mol/L	Under 7 micro mol/L
Iron	Up to 180 mg/dL	Under 100 mg/dL
C-reactive protein	Up to 4.9 mg/L	Under 2 mg/L
Fibrinogen	Up to 460 mg/dL	Under 300 mg/dL
Tryglycerides	Up to 199 mg/dL	Under 100 mg/dL

OH, AND ONE MORE THING . . . GET YOUR TEETH CHECKED! No matter how much you hate to do it, you'd better get to the dentist. It seems that flossing and regular checkups for periodontal disease can help save your heart. At the year 2000 annual meeting of the American Heart Association, Dr. Efthymios N. Deliargyris of the University of North Carolina at Chapel Hill announced the results of a study he had conducted. It showed that among thirty-eight people who experienced a first heart attack, 85 percent of them had advanced gum disease. They also showed much higher levels of C-reactive protein in their blood than such patients without gum disease. In an article on the EurekAlert website (www.eurekalert.org), Dr. Deliargyris was quoted as saying, "Not only did the heart attack patients with periodontal disease have higher levels of CRP than those without gum disease, but the CRP levels were directly related to the severity of the gum disease. The more severe the gum disease, the higher the CRP levels." The way this seems to work is that when you have periodontal disease, the gum separates from the bone, making it easier for bacteria to be absorbed into the bloodstream. Those bacteria then initiate an inflammatory response, which raises the level of CRP, which then increases the risk of heart attack. So you might want to put down this book for a few minutes and go call your dental hygienist!

Diagnostic Testing Part III

Functional Assessment

According to the *Functional Assessment Resource Manual* of the Great Smokies Diagnostic Laboratory, functional assessments are the primary diagnostic tools for Functional Medicine, designed to enable "early intervention into the improvement of physiological, cognitive/emotional and physical functioning. . . . Ideally, functional medicine focuses on prevention and restoration of efficient physiological function. A central principle of functional medicine is that maintaining optimal function leads to a longer life of optimal health."

And that's what we're all after—optimal health. Traditional medicine patches up the body's failing systems. We demand more than that in the twenty-first century. And most often, it's up to us to get it for ourselves. We can no longer rely on our doctors to tell us everything we need to know. Doctors are not really the ones to blame for this situation. Technology is moving so quickly, and there's only so much information they can absorb for the hundreds of patients they may have. Years ago, there was nowhere for a patient to go to get information about a particular disease or disorder.

But in our High-Tech world, we have almost unlimited information at our fingertips (or mouse tips). In fact, we often end up knowing more than the doctor does about what ails us. The Internet has enabled us to be medical detectives. Remember, though, that the information on the Internet is not regulated; not everything you find is legitimate. You must always check your sources and never follow advice without knowing its basis and scientific reliability.

What this chapter offers is information about staying well, and that includes diagnostic tests that check your wellness levels. You don't have to wait until you get sick to make yourself better. You can learn about these tests yourself and suggest them to your doctor. If your doctor doesn't perform them, you may want to find a Functional Medicine practitioner who will do them for you. These tests allow you to get the bigger picture of your health and where your body may be headed. But you need to know that these tests exist before you can ask for them. Take advantage of the fact that we live in the information age, and don't let ill health come to you by surprise.

The following functional assessments are available from the Great Smokies Diagnostic Laboratory, but you can have similar tests done at different labs. These are six tests that we recommend to cover major body systems (there are, of course, other tests that are available for specific problems):

Test 1: Comprehensive Digestive Stool Analysis (for the gastrointestinal system)

Why do you need it? Poor digestion can lead to:

- gas and bloating

- abdominal pain

- diarrhea

- constipation

- food allergies

- production of toxins

- increased risk of colon cancer

- increased risk of ulcerative colitis

This test takes a comprehensive look at the gastrointestinal tract, with information about digestion, absorption, bacterial balance, yeast overgrowth, inflammation, metabolic activity, and immune function.

Test 2: Amino Acids Analysis (for nutritional deficits)

Why do you need it? Amino acid imbalances can lead to:

- mood and behavioral disorders

- hormone imbalances

- elevated homocysteine levels

- impaired hepatic detoxification

- food allergies

- zinc and/or magnesium deficiencies

This test looks at deficiencies in amino acids, the building blocks that make up protein in all bodily tissues, including bone, muscle, ligaments, tendons, hair, glands, and organs. Amino acids are also the basic constituents of hormones, enzymes, and neurotransmitters.

Test 3: Adrenocortex Stress Profile (for the hormonal system)

Why do you need it? Excess stress can lead to:

- chronic fatigue

- depression

- panic disorders

- male impotence

- infertility

- PMS

- anorexia nervosa

- sleep disturbances

This test takes a comprehensive look at the endocrine system, especially DHEA and cortisol.

Test 4: Male Hormone Profile (for testosterone levels)

Why do you need it? Below normal testosterone levels can lead to:

- sexual dysfunction and/or impotence

- cardiovascular disease

- loss of bone and muscle strength

- premature aging

- low energy

- sleep disturbances

- poor cognitive function

The male sex hormone influences a lot more than just sexual function, including emotional well-being, cardiovascular health, and cognitive ability. This test measures testosterone levels, as well as DHEA and cortisol.

Test 5: Female Hormone Profile (for estrogen, progesterone, and testosterone)

Why do you need it? Female hormone imbalances can lead to:

- PMS

- menstrual irregularities

- sleep disturbances

- loss of sexual drive

- infertility

- osteoporosis

- endometriosis

- breast cancer

This test takes a comprehensive look at women's hormones, which play an increasing role in their health as they age. Low estrogen levels are associated with stress, headaches, and osteoporosis, while high estrogen levels increase the risk for breast cancer, especially for postmenopausal women. A profile such as this can help you make knowledgeable decisions about such matters as hormone replacement therapy.

Test 6: Comprehensive Cardiovascular Assessment (for the cardiovascular system)

Why do you need it? Elevated cardiovascular markers can lead to:

- arteriosclerosis

- heart attack

- stroke

This assessment test is for cholesterol levels, homocysteine, triglycerides (fatty acids derived from glucose), Lp(a), and C-reactive protein.

There are many places around the country that will perform similar diagnostic testing. Some of them require that you have blood drawn for testing; others rely on a saliva sample.

One place you can turn to for blood testing is The Life Extension Foundation (LEF). They offer dozens of different blood tests, including those for hormone levels (male and female), cancer markers, homocysteine, and fibrinogen. You can contact LEF either by phone or at their website to order blood testing kits. They will send you a list of places in your area where you can have your blood drawn. You then send the samples to LEF, they will send the results back to you, and you can take them to your doctor for help in interpreting those results. Check out the resource guide at the end of the book for their phone number and address, as well as other places that offer various testing services.

One of the newest (and many think most reliable) ways of checking for hormone imbalances is saliva testing. Scientists have known for almost thirty years that hormones could be measured in saliva, but it is only recently that technology has made that possibility a reality.

When hormones are released from various glands into the bloodstream, they are bound to proteins too large to pass into the saliva. However, a small fraction of these hormones (1 to 5 percent) breaks loose from the protein and is then biologically available to its target tissue (breast, uterus, brain, et cetera). It is the free or unbound hormone that gives you a true measure of your hormone levels.

Testing hormone levels is an important aspect of High-Tech health, especially as we age (and especially for women who are approaching menopause). As Ann Louise Gittleman says in her book *Before the Change,* "The result of hormone level tests lets you know immediately if something is seriously out of line. When you know what your hormone level is, you can then seek treatment, if you need it, on an individualized basis."

There are several advantages to saliva testing. You no longer have to go to a doctor's office to have blood drawn or to drop off a urine sample. Having blood drawn can be a stressful event for some people, and may even alter hormone levels, therefore affecting the test results. Saliva testing can be done at home. Hormones are more stable in saliva than they are in blood, so saliva samples can be safely stored at room temperature for at least a week, which means they can be shipped to a laboratory by regular mail (not kept on ice packs like blood samples).

Because you don't need a doctor's prescription or referral for saliva testing, there are many places that offer kits for home use, including the one that Ann Louise Gittleman recommends, Uni Key Health Systems in Bozeman, Montana (see resource guide).

Diagnostic Testing Part IV

High-Tech Scanning

Although scanners have not yet reached the levels of Dr. McCoy's handheld devices, they have come pretty far. Scanners, like X rays, take pictures of your insides. Twenty-first-century scanning devices go deeper and into more detail than any X ray has ever gone before.

High-Tech scanning is still somewhat controversial. That's because it belongs to the new paradigm—these devices are used mainly to catch risk factors and diseases at their earliest stages. In other words, like diagnostic testing, you have these scans done to determine your current state of health and to look for possible trouble spots. Two of the most promising scanners are Electron-Beam Computed Tomography and the 3D CT scan.

Electron-Beam Computed Tomography (EBCT)

This High-Tech scanner is used to detect coronary artery calcification (CAC), or calcium deposits, in the arteries that feed the heart. Strong statistical evidence shows that the presence of calcium deposits often leads to coronary heart disease.

According to the University HeartScan in New York City, the EBCT "has the unique ability to detect and quantify small amounts of calcified plaque in the coronary arteries" and can "predict a person's risk for heart disease—years before symptoms are present." An EBCT can diagnose coronary heart disease before arteries become blocked; conventional tests can only detect calcification when arteries are blocked at least 50 percent.

There are more than 120 diagnostic and medical centers throughout the world that offer this test, which takes approximately eight minutes and costs anywhere from $300 to $600. If a doctor has sent you to get scanned because you have experienced symptoms, such as chest pains, the cost may be covered by insurance. If you want to find out for yourself if you have calcium deposits, you will have to pay for the test yourself.

There is controversy about this diagnostic tool. In June 2000, a committee from the American Heart Association and the American College of Cardiology announced that it would not recommend the test for seemingly "healthy" people—those who had no symptoms and no multiple risk factors, such as high cholesterol, high blood pressure, obesity, diabetes, or family history of heart disease. The committee also cited a 43 percent false positive rate for the test, which then costs patients unnecessary worry and thousands of dollars in follow-up tests. They did acknowledge that the test would benefit those who had some symptoms and/or risk factors for heart disease, by measuring the amount of calcium deposits that were present. In many diagnostic centers, the same technology is being used to scan the lungs for nodules and smoke-related damage.

3D CT Scan

A new technology that is even more futuristic than the EBCT is the 3D CT scan, or what I like to call a "virtual autopsy." The difference is that you're still alive when they do it.

It is just what it sounds like—a three-dimensional computerized journey through your own body from the neck to the pelvis. The technology was developed in the mid-1980s as a heart-scanning device, but has now expanded to include the entire torso. The 3D scan can be used to detect abnormalities and disease throughout the body. It can augment mammography in the early detection of breast cancer and detect signs of prostate disease. It can detect early signs of osteoporosis, aneurysms, vascular disease, cancer, benign tumors, and kidney stones and gallstones. It is also used to conduct a noninvasive "virtual colonoscopy" that, according to a 1999 article in the *New England Journal of Medicine*, has "similar efficacy for the detection of polyps" that are likely to be cancerous. One of the first centers in the nation to offer this diagnostic tool is the Health View Center for Preventive Medicine in Newport Beach, California, run by radiologist Dr. Harvey Eisenberg. The clinic has scanned many thousands of patients and has thousands more on its waiting list. Critics say that the scanning is too expensive (the test runs about $700 and is not covered by most insurance). They cite the same objection as for the EBCT—that ambiguous results often lead to unnecessary, invasive, and expensive follow-up tests.

Eisenberg responded to these objections in an article for *USA Today*, noting that "medicine today often chases after a disease with treatments when it's already too late to reverse the damage to the body. . . . By the time a disease is diagnosed . . . doctors can only try to 'catch up.' That isn't right. Medicine has to change its paradigm from being reactive to proactive. Crisis management doesn't work."

My Own Fantastic Voyage

When I heard about this new technology, I had to see it for myself. So I took a trip out to California to have my own 3D scan done. It was quite an eye-opening experience.

The anticipation was probably the hardest part. What would they find inside these "old" bones of mine? I've been taking care of myself fairly well for many years—but those years were preceded by teenage and young adult years of typical recklessness. How much damage had those years wrought?

The experience of the scan itself was quite simple. You lie on your back, fully dressed, in an open CT scanner for a little more than fifteen minutes. Then comes the mostly fascinating, partly scary aftermath, where you sit down with one of Health View's professionals and play back the results. It is peculiar looking at your own insides, dissected organ by organ.

We started by looking at the heart and arteries, which, amazingly, showed no plaque buildup. Usually a person of my age (forty-nine at the time) will exhibit some plaque. The fact that I have none tells me that my years of Paleotech nutrition and fitness, plus my use of antioxidants and supplements, kept my arterial passageways clear.

There were other areas that were of more concern, although thankfully we did not find anything serious or life threatening. I have a very small calcium deposit in my right kidney, which is considered to be very common. There was a slight enlargement of the prostate consistent with my age. That was of particular concern to me, because my father had prostate cancer years ago. I have no signs of cancer, but I need to be sure and so I have my PSA tested every year. When we looked at my bones, there was some deterioration and inflammatory damage in my lower spine and hips, probably due to twenty-five years of being a runner and a marathoner. I expected that. I didn't expect what I saw in my lungs.

I started smoking when I was sixteen years old and quickly began to smoke at least a pack a day, sometimes two packs a day. At the age of twenty, I suffered a partially collapsed lung. Even that wasn't enough to shake the habit; all I could think about was waiting for my two-week recovery period to end so that I could have

A TRUE DIAGNOSTIC TALE Not long ago a new client came into my office, a seventy-year-old gentleman (whom I will call William) who appeared to be in very good health. He was seeking some nutritional counseling. He brought with him records of "complete" blood work he got from his doctor. His doctor had not checked for heart markers like homocysteine. PSA levels had not been checked. His doctor had told him only that perhaps he "needed to slow down a bit." I sent him to the University HeartScan. They found extensive calcium deposits in the major vessels. His heart was enlarged. They found that he had two gallstones. William is a wealthy man, who went to the "best" doctors. Even his cardiologist did not pick up these abnormalities. I had his homocysteine level checked. It was 18. Even the "standard reference ranges" only go up to 15. This man was in serious danger of heart disease, heart attack, and/or stroke, and none of his doctors had discovered it. Using these new diagnostic tools, he has now adjusted his diet and lifestyle, and is taking proper supplementation to address his condition. He was beyond indignant that even the "best" doctors had not recommended these tests. He is now, needless to say, a vocal proponent of High-Tech diagnostic tools.

another cigarette. Finally, at the age of twenty-four, after I went to the emergency room suffering from severe chest pains, I gave up the "evil weed."

Here I was, twenty-five years later, and to my shock, my lungs still showed signs of damage, albeit quite small. There were tiny black patches in the lower left-hand corner that Dr. Eisenberg said were emphysema cells. "Nothing else but tobacco causes that kind of destruction," he said. I was lucky, he said, because there were no signs of cancer and, even with that small shadow from the past, my lungs were actually healthy.

Right now, a 3D CT scan is far from standard practice. But it took almost twenty years before mammograms were considered standard practice, and now at least 15 percent of women who would have died are saved because of it. It may take fifteen or twenty years for these new High-Tech diagnostic tools to be accepted.

Where Do We Go from Here?

Unfortunately, there are thousands of diseases that afflict mankind, so finding ways to detect all of them may never be possible. However, new breakthroughs are being seen every day, especially regarding two of mankind's most dreaded diseases, Alzheimer's and cancer.

Alzheimer's One breakthrough appeared in the September 2000 issue of the *American Journal of Psychiatry* in an article titled "Olfactory deficits in patients with mild cognitive impairment predict Alzheimer's follow-up." In other words, a simple scratch-and-sniff test may be a predictor for the disease. Scientists had known for years that people with Alzheimer's tend to show impairments in their ability to detect and identify odors. So a group from Columbia University, led by Dr. D. P. Devanand, wanted to find out if an impaired sense of smell preceded the disease. They studied ninety men and women, nineteen of whom did poorly on the smell test. Sixteen of those nineteen went on to develop Alzheimer's. Studies are now being done with larger groups of people.

Using this test, we may be able to tell who is a likely candidate to develop the disease. Although that information may not lead to an instant cure (there is no known cure yet), it will certainly help scientists in their efforts to find one.

Cancer   There are probably thousands of studies going on at any one time all over the world, trying to find tumor markers, or signs in the body that will aid in the prediction and early diagnosis of cancer. One of the major problems is that there is not just one disease called *cancer*. Every type of cancer behaves differently and therefore may have different predictors. Taking a PSA test for prostate cancer, for instance, will not tell you whether or not you have brain or liver cancer.

That said, the research into tumor markers continues. The National Cancer Institute defines tumor markers as "... substances that can often be detected in higher-than-normal amounts in the blood, urine, or body tissues of some patients with certain types of cancer. Tumor markers are produced either by the tumor itself or by the body in response to the presence of certain benign conditions." The NCI also notes that currently, tumor markers are being used mainly to assess a cancer's "... response to a treatment and to check for recurrence. Scientists continue to study these uses of tumor markers as well as their potential role in the early detection and diagnosis of cancer."

In many ways, diagnostic testing is the future of the Healthy High-Tech Body. If we can detect the onset of disease long before it actually manifests itself, we can take steps to prevent its occurrence or drastically reduce its consequences. In that sense, the twenty-first century has begun with a bang: the Human Genome Project. Scientists have already identified thousands of genes in which defects can cause disease. In some cases, that knowledge has already led to new approaches for curing those diseases.

In an article for the *Seattle Post-Intelligencer*, Lee Hartwell, director of the Fred Hutchinson Cancer Research Center, stated that "the difficulty—and this is the hardest thing for the public to understand—is all we ever will be able to say is there is a certain probability of getting a disease. Say, over the next five years, your chances are such and such. But if we know that 1 percent of a population is susceptible to a certain disease, then we can monitor much more closely for early appearance of symptoms and control the disease at an earlier stage. That will be the greatest payoff."

Hartwell also noted that what the genome project is teaching us about disease is complicated by the fact that no two humans are alike, which means that we all respond differently to different treatments. However, "the promise in this is that it will be the first step in individualized medicine." The assumption today is that if something works for me, it will work for you as well. The knowledge of our High-Tech future will enable us to diagnose, measure, and treat disease on a purely case-by-case basis.

Pillar 4
The Body Beautiful

Let's face it. We want to live long, healthy lives.

We just don't want to look old while we're doing it. Don't worry. The past few years have brought major advances in what we know about our skin, our nails, our teeth, our hair. There are exciting new products and treatments available today that can help us look our best for tomorrow.

As you'll see in chapter 11, "Looking Good Longer," beauty is definitely more than skin deep. It starts, as do all the Healthy High-Tech Body protocols, with proper nutrition, exercise, sleep, and stress reduction. There are no overnight creams that will make you look twenty years younger and solve all your beauty problems in one treatment.

There is, however, a wide variety of products and treatments from which to choose. And you'll have the benefit of the knowledge and science of three great authorities on skin and hair—Dr. Nicholas Perricone, Dr. Stephen Bosniak, and Dr. Peter Proctor.

In chapter 12, "Hair Today, Hair Tomorrow," you'll be glad to learn that there is hope (albeit no cure) for those who are "follicly impaired." There's much that you can do to prevent hair loss, and in some cases regrow hair that's already gone (think of it—no more plugs, no more combovers!). Again, there is no easy answer, but there are a lot of options you should know about.

And what would the beautiful body be without fitness? We've already discussed many of the incredible benefits of a regular exercise program. "High-Level Fitness" takes you one step further, into the science and fitness of the future. After all, you have to be physically fit in order to take the best possible advantage of the years that the Healthy High-Tech Body just may add on to your life.

11 Looking Good Longer

Cosmeceuticals for skin, nails, and teeth

Remember the film *Death in Venice?* Dirk Bogarde starred as the lovestruck lead in Venice in the early 1900s. Bogarde, in pursuit of a much younger lover, is desperate to improve his aging appearance. There is an unforgettable scene in a barbershop. There Bogarde sits, getting his hair dyed and his face made up. The end product (as you see him in search of his love interest) is tragic. The makeup is obvious. His attempts at looking younger are simply grotesque. At the end of the film, Bogarde is seen lying on a beach as his new look begins to melt away in the sun. It's achingly painful.

That film was made in 1971, based on a story written in the 1930s. Things have not changed very much since then; we still believe that youth is god. We are not much different in our pursuits today when it comes to looking good. There are lots of people who put all their faith in hair dye and makeup, in cosmetic surgery or liposuction, yet are not willing to put in the work to generate healthy tissue. The results are often not at all what they hoped they would be.

If you follow the suggestions in this chapter and the next one, you will probably look younger. You will definitely look healthier and more vibrant. This chapter is about beauty in the sense that it is about achieving your best looks, how to have the best-looking skin, nails, smile, and hair you can have, using twenty-first-century knowledge and technology. What is currently available to enhance your beauty is dazzling. There are many important things to consider that will allow you to maintain your "beauty" effortlessly. *That's not to say you'll have the skin of a baby at eighty, or the hair of a twenty-year-old, but you will have skin and hair that reflect the look of health.*

This is a mix-and-match chapter; use all the strategies laid out for you to rejuvenate your healthy appearance. The look you want is not just a matter of taking care of your external self. It's a result of how well your internal biochemistry is nourished. It begins with the quality of your diet and ends with the kind and quality of products you use externally. It means using all these varied tools and developing the strategies that will let you control wrinkling, loose skin, damaged nails, deteriorating teeth and gums.

There's nothing wrong with enhancing your looks via cosmetic surgery and liposuction; those are personal choices. For some people, they may be the right choices. But even they won't *maintain* a youthful appearance unless you back them up *by controlling the combined damaging forces of inflammation, glycation, and free-radical damage.*

There are countless products and services on the market today that promise to perform miracles. But unless they can control the combined damage of inflammation, glycation, and free radicals, they wind up being cosmetic Band-Aids. Even so, we've come a long way from using tea bags under our eyes and sticking our heads in cold buckets of ice to get the "puffiness" out. We've entered into a whole new era of personal enhancement.

What Makes Us Look Old?

It's the great paradox of our youth-obsessed society: how do you continue to look young even as you get older? The fact is, we all play a role in accelerating the aging of our own tissue. Some people are simply genetically endowed with great beauty by cultural standards, which is usually most obvious when they are young. When we're young, we're still pumping out plenty of growth factors, enzymes, and hormones that keep everything looking firm and fit. You stay out all night, splash some cold water on your face the next day, pop two aspirin, swallow them with a cup of coffee, and keep going, looking not a day older. Try that at fifty, and you wind up looking seventy. The older you are, the less effort it takes to speed up looking bad.

Stress hormones wear down your looks and begin to kill off your hair follicles. The puffiness around your eyes becomes a permanent fixture along with puffiness around your gut and everywhere else. Some people look this way after the age of fifty, some at thirty or thirty-five. The negative effects of the pursuit of "master of the universe" status take their toll on all of us—it just starts earlier for some than for others.

In my own youth, I enjoyed a career in fashion photography. I worked with many models of breathtaking beauty. Some of them are still gorgeous today. But models don't necessarily take great care to maintain their beauty. I recently ran into a model friend I had not seen in years. She was just about unrecognizable. She still clutched a cigarette in one hand, as she had when I had known her all those years ago. She hadn't just aged, she had worn out her looks. In fact, smoking is one of the most damaging habits you can have, not only in terms of health, but in terms of how you look. An article by Paul Brodish for the American Council on Science and Health titled "The Irreversible Effects of Cigarette Smoking" revealed why people who smoke for many years get that distinctive "smoker's face": "Smoking causes premature facial wrinkling through vasoconstriction of the capillaries of the face (vasoconstriction decreases the flow of oxygen and nutrients to facial tissue). The effect of this reduced blood flow is visible in deep crow's feet radiating from the corners of the eyes and pale, grayish, wrinkled skin on the cheeks. These effects may emerge after as few as five years of smoking and are largely irreversible."

And, according to Dr. Nicholas Perricone, author of *The Wrinkle Cure* and my favorite authority in the field of reversing skin aging, "there is a 15 to 20 year difference in the appearances of smokers versus nonsmokers."

Of course, tobacco is not the only factor that affects your looks. Everything that goes into or onto your body, as well as how you treat it, affects the way you look. Some other influential factors include:

- whether or not you're properly hydrated

- how much sun you get (too much, not enough)

- the quality of your diet

- the external products you use

- the volume of recreational damage you inflict on your body

Multiply these factors by how well you manage stress and how much sleep you get and you have the equation for your aging appearance. So what are the various kinds of damage that occur to the skin, and what can you do prevent and correct them?

Inflammation, Free Radicals, Glycation, and Your Aging Skin

As I've pointed out throughout this book, one of the largest problems we face as we age is inflammatory damage to our bodies. There is a highly inflammatory compound in our cells called nuclear factor kappa B or NFkB. Any number of things can turn up the volume on the production and activity of NFkB, including poor nutrition and too much sun exposure. Free radicals start the whole process.

Free radicals are unstable oxygen molecules that are produced when oxygen interacts with organic matter. The most obvious example of free-radical damage and how quickly it operates is when you cut open an apple and place it on a counter. It will rapidly begin to turn brown as oxygen interacts with the organic tissue of the apple and free radicals are being generated. We're spoiling in the same way the apple does, but at a slower rate. In our bodies, free radicals are generated by sunlight, tobacco, carcinogens, excitotoxins, pollutants of all kinds, and highly modified foods such as deep-fried anything.

Free radicals stimulate the production of the NFkB inflammatory compound, which in turn switches on the production of additional tissue-damaging compounds, resulting in what is called "micro-scarring." Produce enough of these micro-scars and you have a wrinkle. This kind of subclinical inflammation takes place below our visual radar; it's a sort of ever-accumulating stealth damage that increases as we age.

"What many people don't understand," says Dr. Nicholas Perricone, "is that free radicals do very little direct damage to our skin. Free radicals have a life of a nanosecond. They're not long-lived enough to do a lot of damage. But free radicals do trigger an inflammatory response. They kick off a chain of chemical events that produces a domino effect that can last minutes, hours, days, weeks, or months.

"I've been talking about this since the late 1980s. Whenever I looked at aging skin under a microscope, there was always an inflammatory component present. Without inflammation, aging doesn't go forward. You can even have skin affected by overexposure to the sun; yet, if there isn't inflammation present it doesn't do the extensive damage you see clinically. *In my opinion, inflammation is at the center of the whole problem of aging!*"

In addition to free-radical and inflammatory damage, you add in the damage that occurs from *glycosylation*. Glycosylation occurs when sugar molecules bind to collagen molecules and make them stiffen; in other words, the overconsumption of any kind of sugar creates the structures that are the signs of aging. As you know from earlier chapters, glycosylation causes *lipofuscion* to occur, creating the browning of your skin. This happens when you get the cross linkage of your collagen, making your skin inflexible and prone to discoloration, producing visible brown spots (that also accumulate "invisibly" on your brain).

The Ground Rules
for Great Skin and Hair

What can you do about all this damage that is taking place inside your body? You can follow the ground rules below.

Ground Rule One

Follow the eating guidelines in the Paleotech Diet. You know from chapter 2 that imbalances in your diet can produce inflammation via the overproduction of insulin. Too much insulin present in your blood (because of too many carbohydrates and too much sugar consumption) causes the overproduction of harmful eicosanoids, which causes inflammation. Take control of your diet and you improve your health and your looks. A diet rich in omega-3 fatty acids and naturally occurring antioxidants found in fruits and vegetables helps to reduce inflammation.

Ground Rule Two

Sunbathe, don't sunburn. Overexposure to the sun and UV light can damage more than your appearance: it can cause skin cancer. Remember this: a tan is not a sign of health. It is a sign that skin has been damaged by ultraviolet radiation. Also remember that skin cancer is very slow to develop; the sunburn you receive this week could become skin cancer in twenty years. Some researchers have estimated that *one serious sunburn can increase your risk of skin cancer by as much as 50 percent.* There really are no High-Tech preventions for this. There are several things you can do, however. First, use a high-quality sunscreen of at least SPF 15 or higher (and if it contains alpha lipoic acid, even better). Second, reapply sunscreen every two hours, even on cloudy days. Third, wear clothing that covers your body and shades your face. And fourth, minimize your exposure to the sun between the hours of 10:00 A.M. and 3:00 P.M.

Ground Rule Three

Use nutraceuticals, in particular alpha lipoic acid, MSM, and silica.

Alpha lipoic acid Considered the "universal" antioxidant, alpha lipoic acid boosts levels of glutathione in all cells, exhibits antioxidant activity in almost all tissues of the body, and improves the antioxidant functionality of vitamin C, vitamin E, and coenzyme Q_{10}. It reduces inflammation, pumps up the immune system, and helps the human body knit together tissue injuries. Alpha lipoic acid is known to fight free radicals in any part of the cell and even in the spaces between them. Here's the neat part: it also works as a powerful anti-inflammatory by preventing the activation of NFkB. This in turn blocks the cells from making pro-inflammatory compounds that accelerate aging. If NFkB is already activated, alpha lipoic acid will round up the free radicals that are generated by the inflammatory compounds.

An additional feature of alpha lipoic acid is that it signals tissue-repairing compounds, including one called transcription factor AP-1, to begin working. Alpha lipoic acid allows AP-1 to "digest" damaged collagen, resulting in the elimination and erasure of wrinkles. It also appears that alpha lipoic acid can protect against glycation by blocking the attachment of sugar to protein. It may reverse glycation damage and protect collagen from the toxic effects of sugar. Recommended dosage is between 10 and 100 milligrams daily.

MSM MSM (which has been mentioned several times in this book because of its myriad benefits) is also effective in its ability to support healthy collagen synthesis. MSM is a form of sulfur critical for building healthy ligaments, bone, muscle tissue, and, yes, great skin and hair. MSM can be taken orally or applied in cream and is an essential nutrient for the maintenance of beauty. The primary protein of hair—keratin—is composed of two building blocks made up of MSM, cysteine, and methionine. Recommended dosage is 500 milligrams (minimum) to 3 grams a day.

Silica This essential nutrient has been around forever as a supplement recommended for healthy hair. It is required for maintaining healthy bones, nails, skin, and teeth. Collagen, tooth enamel, and even our gums benefit from bioavailable silica. It is found primarily in nature in a plant called horsetail. My recommendation is Silica Gel by Body Essential. Take one teaspoon a day, in juice, water, or a shake. Use Silica Gel in combination with MSM for at least three months to see great improvement in the quality of your hair, skin, and nails.

Ground Rule Four

Use high-quality cosmeceuticals. The term *cosmeceutical,* coined by Dr. Nicholas Perricone, refers to a type of skin product that provides added benefit to your skin, above and beyond what a commercial cosmetic or moisturizer can provide. Cosmeceuticals, applied externally, incorporate nutrient antioxidants in very novel ways that can impede and even repair the damage to skin cells that comes with aging. They are not considered medications and therefore not regulated by the FDA.

It's important to point out that antioxidant "dense" products—used for protecting and repairing skin damage—work better when applied topically than when ingested. A study reported in *Skin and Allergy News* confirmed that antioxidants added to sunscreens provided even greater protection from solar radiation, inhibiting more lines and wrinkles and maintaining greater skin elasticity and thickness than sunscreen without antioxidants.

There are many skin conservation products available today, some more effective than others. Two product lines stand out because of their use of cutting-edge, scientifically based ingredients.

REJUVENEX BY LIFE EXTENSION FOUNDATION

One of the most effective ingredients of Rejuvenex products is hyaluronic acid (HA), which was the focus of an interesting study. It seems there's a village outside of Tokyo, Japan, called Yuziri Hara. It's also been called the "village of long life." Everybody in Yuziri Hara lives to a ripe old age, with almost no cancer, diabetes, or Alzheimer's disease. More than 10 percent of the population is over eighty-five years of age, ten times the American norm. These villagers are not necessarily paragons of virtue; many have smoked cigarettes for most of their lives and/or worked outdoors in the sun without sunblock or protection. Yet they remain reasonably fit and exhibit soft and smooth skin at age ninety. Scientists have yet to discover their secret. But signs point to their diet, rich in omega-3 fatty acids (of course); specifically there is "something" in this diet that stimulates the human body to produce hyaluronic acid, which aging bodies typically lose.

HA helps to keep human cells "thriving" and joints lubricated (there's an injectable form used to treat osteoarthritis), retain tissue hydration, and protect the skin by keeping it smooth and elastic. HA has been shown to be effective in tissue reconstruction and healing wounds. When applied externally, it can soften facial lines and improve the firmness and elasticity of skin.

HA is not the only unusual (and unusually effective) ingredient in Rejuvenex. It has twenty-six active ingredients used to control inflammation and to signal the skin to increase the synthesis of healthy new collagen. Rejuvenex works to suppress free-radical damage to the skin and inhibit mechanisms that age skin prematurely (including those involved in UV radiation damage from the sun). This is a High-Tech multitasking product line that's a requisite for maintaining the integrity of your skin.

DR. NICHOLAS PERRICONE'S WRINKLE CURE

For the serious devotee of extraordinary skin health and appearance, this line of products is the standard of excellence. Here we have alpha lipoic acid, DMAE, vitamin C, and vitamin E being used in very new and powerful ways. This line of cosmeceuticals is made up of five components:

- alpha lipoic acid

- vitamin C esters

- DMAE

- tocotrienols, a high-potency form of vitamin E

- alpha-hydroxy and beta-hydroxy 5

Alpha lipoic acid. Since ALA extends the effectiveness of antioxidants such as vitamin C, vitamin E, and glutathione, it offers extra skin protection. This is a triple-whammy ingredient—it helps suppress free-radical damage and prevent inflammatory damage and control glycation. ALA visibly reduces swelling, especially around the eyes, and can also reduce the numbers of enlarged pores on skin (a condition that rarely responds to other skin treatments). It is also useful in minimizing rosacea, a skin problem characterized by redness, bumps, and broken blood vessels on the face.

Vitamin C esters. Vitamin C is one of the most frequently studied and applied antioxidants under the sun (pun intended). It has been proven to help prevent heart disease and some forms of cancer and strengthen the immune system. It turns out that vitamin C is also essential for the production of collagen, and it is a prominent factor in reducing inflammation. It accomplishes this reduction by reducing the production of *arachidonic acid,* which is a bad eicasonoid that causes everything from inflammatory pain to heart disease. Arachidonic acid is also involved in the production of micro-scarring, which leads to wrinkling.

Although there are a number of vitamin C products that work well on skin, the one developed by Nicholas Perricone is completely nonirritating and is easily absorbed. It is especially good for sun-damaged skin, penetrating the thin membranes that encase a cell. This offers your skin cells the maximum protection against free-radical damage at the point at which they do the greatest harm, *the outer lining of the cell.* The "ester" form (vitamin C combined with a fat called palmitic acid) is the most effective method for delivery to your tissues. This product is best used for erasing fine lines and wrinkles on severely sun-damaged skin; for sagging skin that is losing its firmness due to lost or damaged collagen; and, as stated, for inflamed, sunburned, and irritated skin.

DMAE. This is a powerful neurotransmitter precursor that the brain uses to improve focus and clarity of mind, alertness, and memory. DMAE also protects cell membranes against degradation, considered one of the prime mechanisms of aging. When used externally, it produces a firming effect—you might even call it an instant facelift. Within twenty to thirty minutes of using DMAE, you can see an improvement in skin tone, with a tighter, more youthful look that lasts for hours. It also appears that the long-term use of DMAE can help permanently increase the firmness of the skin, and it is used on the face and the neck. This fast-acting, effective cosmeceutical is used in several products formulated by Dr. Perricone. I recommend them often for many of my clients in entertainment who require a *rapid* improvement in their faces for an imminent appearance.

Tocotrienol vitamin E. Some studies suggest that this palm oil–derived vitamin E may be up to forty times more potent than standard types of vitamin E (usually in a form called a tocopherol, which you can pick up at your local health food store) for protection against elevated cholesterol and the plaque formation common in atherosclerosis. Studies also indicate that this form of vitamin E may be more effective for skin and hair. It can be used to make hair shinier, increase sunscreen effectiveness, and heal redness and scaling in severely dry and damaged skin. The secret may lie in the chemical structure and action of this form of vitamin E. It completely disperses in a cell membrane, moving about rapidly and neutralizing free radicals far more effectively than standard vitamin E.

Alpha-hydroxy and beta-hydroxy 5. Alpha-hydroxy acids (AHA) were developed for people who wanted the benefits of Retin-A without its negative side effects. Alpha-hydroxy acids are naturally occurring acids, derived from sugars in plants like sugar cane, grapes, and citrus fruits. They work by dissolving the substances that hold dead skin together, making it easier for them to slough off. In high doses, AHA is an effective chemical peel. Used in low doses, AHA appears to be effective in reducing signs of aging skin produced by too much sun and other environmental factors.

For the complete program of skin repair and efficiency, read Dr. Perricone's informative book, *The Wrinkle Cure*. For the complete line of products, go to www.nvperriconemd.com, where you'll find the various formulations and a helpful FAQ section. My Healthy High-Tech Body recommendations, although they may vary for you depending on your skin type and particular needs, include:

- **Alpha Lipoic Face Firming Activator w/NTP Complex:** this is a great resurfacing product, including DMAE, ALA, glycolic acid.

- **Vitamin C Ester Amine Complex Face Lift w/NTP:** great for accentuating your facial contours, including vitamin C ester plus DMAE.

- **Alpha Lipoic Body Toning Lotion SPF 15 w/NTP:** great to use all over your body; for improving tone and firmness, it includes ALA, DMAE, plus UVA and UVB protection.

High-Tech Skin Care Options: Injectable Hyaluronic Acid, Botox, and Laser Surgery

Hyaluronic Acid Injections

Hyaluronic acid (HA) has been used in cataract surgery for over twenty-five years, injected into the eyeball to keep it from collapsing during surgery. It is also used to lubricate the joints of arthritic patients, marketed under the name Hyaloronan.

Recently, injectable HA has begun to be used as a wrinkle filler. Traditionally, collagen (or your own fat) was injected into the deep folds on either side of your nostrils to lessen these lines. A newer synthetic form of HA called Restylene, and even newer generations such as Macrolene and Perlane (which are being used overseas and are quite popular in Brazil right now), will likely be the next advancement in addressing these facial "imperfections," providing better quality and longer-lasting results. These versions of HA are nonanimal derivatives and pose fewer problems in terms of allergic reactions and inflammation.

Botox

Several years ago, I heard about a doctor at the Equinox Fitness Spa in New York City who was doing some great work getting rid of the tired, worn-out look that people get when they've been working and worrying for way too many years. Dr. Stephen Bosniak was successfully eliminating brow furrows and crow's feet, leaving patients looking as though they'd just gotten back from a week in the Caribbean.

It turned out that Dr. Bosniak had participated in the clinical trials of Botox in the early 1980s and was one of the first to use it in his practice. Botox is an extract of botulinum toxin A. This was the pathogen that caused the Black Plague during the Middle Ages; it is probably best known as the cause of botulism food poisoning. Harnessed by modern medicine, it is used to treat a host of medical conditions, such as eye spasms, central nervous system disorders, and excessive muscle contractions. Quite by accident, it was found to reduce wrinkles and crow's feet.

HOW BOTOX WORKS Botox actually works by causing paralysis. It blocks nerve signals transmitted from the brain to the muscle; specifically, it inhibits the release of acetylcholine from the nerve. In 1989, the FDA approved Botox to correct eyelid spasms and eye muscle problems. Doctors then noticed that after treatment, patients also experienced disappearance of wrinkles in the eye area. They then began using it to reduce frown lines between the eyebrows, crow's feet, and forehead lines. When injected in the forehead and eye area, it prevents patients from frowning or squinting, thus protecting against progressive worsening of lines and wrinkles in these areas.

According to Dr. Bosniak, an ophthalmic surgeon, "Botox is one of the safest and easiest procedures to incorporate in a beautifying program. There are many people for whom a face-lift is not an option, either in terms of affordability, or the time to recover. Yet you can come into our office and get a wonderfully aesthetically pleasing result. Many of our patients come in for Botox treatments two or three times a year. And in the right hands you can produce a very natural-looking effect."

Laser Skin Resurfacing

One of the most advanced treatments available for reversing the effects of aging on your skin is laser skin resurfacing, the use of short-pulse, high-peak power lasers to vaporize the epidermis. Damaged or aging skin is carefully removed layer by layer with a high-energy beam of laser light.

For many years, the process of skin resurfacing has been done using chemical solutions. In what is known as a chemical peel, a solution is applied to the skin, which causes it to separate and eventually peel off. The new skin is smoother and less wrinkled than the old. You have several options when it comes to chemical peels: you can use a light peel made up of *glycolic acid*, fruit-derived chemicals that act to remove the top layer of dead skin cells on your face, hands, or body; *beta lift* peels, which go deeper into the oil-secreting glands; and *trichloroacetic acid (TCA)* peels, which can go much deeper to correct pigmentation, discoloration, and extreme sun damage. The type you choose (in consultation with your doctor) depends on the extent of the damage you are trying to correct. Chemical peels, however, create a reaction similar to mild to severe sunburn and can involve redness, scaling, and blisters. Recovery times vary depending on the intensity of the peel.

Laser skin resurfacing was developed as an alternative to chemical peels. According to the National Skin Center, "Laser resurfacing can duplicate the results of chemical peels. . . . Compared to other methods of skin resurfacing, laser resurfacing has several advantages. It is bloodless and cleaner. . . . There is less postoperative pain, less swelling and bruising resulting in quicker patient recovery."

EYE SURGERY WITHOUT SCALPELS Dr. Bosniak and his partner, Dr. Marian Zilka, have also pioneered the use of the carbon dioxide laser for eye lifts and eye surgery. "The eyelids are a series of unique structures," says Dr. Bosniak. "They're the most delicate structures in the body. They have the thinnest skin in the body. They have their own muscles. Each eyelid has 5 layers of thin tissue, a series of three muscles. And it blinks 100 times a minute. Think about using a scalpel or scissors in this area! We haven't used them in over 7 years. We use a variety of lasers instead. You can be much more accurate with the laser. There is virtually no bleeding, which means the surgery goes by more quickly because you're not stopping bleeding and cutting blood vessels all the time. And the patient will heal faster because there will be less damage to the tissue."

The precision of the laser vaporizes wrinkles and other defects while uncovering healthy skin. There are currently two types of lasers used in skin resurfacing: carbon dioxide and Erbium. While carbon dioxide lasers can be used for even severe skin problems, Erbium lasers are the latest advancement for treatment of less severe age- and sun-damaged skin. The Erbium laser gently vaporizes damaged skin layer by layer. Some studies have also shown that Erbium laser treatments stimulate the production of collagen, smoothing and firming the skin.

The Continuum of External Skin Care

Many aging baby boomers considering ways to make themselves appear younger go right to a plastic surgeon for a face-lift consultation. This is not the place to start. Of course, the best idea is to have taken care of your skin from day one, but most of us have not been that vigilant. But even if you're suddenly realizing at the age of forty that you'd better take better care of yourself, you don't have to head off to the operating room. Consider your options along a continuum of care that can begin at any age and be followed for the rest of your life.

Start with diet, exercise, rest, and stress reduction. Introduce cosmeceuticals. Then, if necessary, move along the continuum treatment line, from least invasive to most invasive, which is a full face-lift. Note that these treatments also work well in combination with each other.

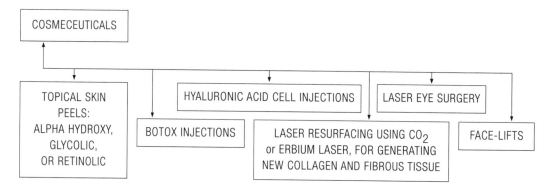

Nail Care: The Long and Short of It

Your nails say a lot about you. They not only broadcast your grooming habits, but also can signal serious disorders in your body.

Nails are made of a protein known as keratin, also found in skin and hair. It's also the same tough protein that's found in birds' beaks, animals' claws, and turtles' shells.

Your nails can reveal much about your overall health:

NAIL PROBLEM	POSSIBLE CAUSE
Small white spots	Zinc deficiency
White nails	Liver disease
Extra-large lunula (half-moon)	Overactive thyroid
Missing lunula	Underactive thyroid
Red or deep pink color	Heart irregularities
Yellow, thickened nail	Lung disease or diabetes
Pale nail bed (skin beneath the nail)	Anemia

Since skin and nails are made of the same substance, the same nutraceuticals that are good for your skin are good for your nails: alpha lipoic acid, MSM, and silica. Other supplements for nail health include: biotin (a colorless, crystalline, water-soluble B complex vitamin also found in egg yolks, beef liver, peanuts, cauliflower, and mushrooms); calcium; vitamin C; vitamin E; and herbs rich in silica, including horsetail, nettle, and oatstraw. An excellent cosmeceutical for nail health is **CP Nail Renewal**, which contains copper peptides and Retinol, available from Skin Biology (see resource guide).

SOME FASCINATING FACTS ABOUT NAILS

- Your nails grow continuously throughout your lifetime, one half to one millimeter per week.
- It takes six to seven months for your fingernail to grow from the root to the fingertip.
- Toenails grow at about half the rate of fingernails.
- Nails grow faster in warm weather than in cold weather.
- Nails grow faster on your dominant hand.
- Men's nails grow faster than women's.
- The lunula—the white, half moon–shaped area at the base of the nail—varies in each finger in each person and disappears as we get older.

Your Twenty-First-Century Smile

The first known dentist was a man named Hesi-Re, who was chief "toothist" to the pharaohs around 3000 B.C. The first known prescription for oral hygiene comes from ancient Assyria-Babylonia and was intended to remove film, whiten discolored teeth, and prevent bad breath. It was a mixture of "salt of Akkad, ammi, Lolium, and pine turpentine." These ingredients were to be mixed together, applied to the teeth, and rubbed with a finger. Then the mouth was to be rinsed with a mixture of "kurunnu-beer, oil and honey."

We've come a long way since kurunnu-beer and honey. In fact, dentistry appears to be on the verge of an exponential change, with giant leaps in everything from diagnostic tools to regenerating teeth. Here are a few of the things we can look forward to in the next decade:

- Current advances in oral microbiology have led to the development of new time-release products. One, Atridox, is a time-release gel for the antibiotic doxycycline. It's injected directly into the pockets that lie between the teeth and the gums and releases the antibiotic over a period of seven days. There's also a device called the Perio-Chip, a wafer that's placed in the gum pocket and releases chlorhexidine antiseptic for about a week. This is useful for reducing the amount of bacteria in the gum line.

- Leery of too many X rays? Mouth cams may soon make that a thing of the past. Tiny cameras are being developed to take video pictures of each tooth, magnified up to twenty times. Digital cameras will be able to create before-and-after images so that patients can see how cosmetic dentistry might change their looks. And a Texas company is developing a tiny camera that could be placed between the tooth and the gum to find and remove bacteria in areas previously accessible only through surgery.

- Regenerative dentistry will become a specialization in the near future. We will soon have the capability to stimulate "tooth growth factors" and regenerate teeth. A dentist and biochemist named William V. Giannobile of the University of Michigan at Ann Arbor has used a viral shell "impregnated" with the gene for human epidermal growth factor and injected it into the gums of pigs. The virus found its way into the pig's gum cell DNA and produced growth factors for four days. Eventually, dentists will be able to custom-grow teeth from cells in a laboratory and use them to replace lost teeth or to grow new ligaments to hold loose teeth in place.

- Bone grafts to hold implanted teeth will become unnecessary. New cements, including one called BoneSource already in existence, are being developed that will not only anchor implanted teeth in place, but will stimulate the body to grow new bone where it is needed.

- New materials are being developed for fillings—materials that would react to bacteria in the mouth and release decay-neutralizers to stop problems before they start.

GIVE YOUR TEETH A TEA BREAK Studies show that oolong and green teas may keep your teeth healthy by reducing the amount of plaque-causing bacteria in your mouth. Both types of tea contain polyphenols, which appear to inhibit the formation of bacteria that promote cavities.

The dentist of the future will likely be capable of diagnosing a myriad of diseases by the state and condition of your teeth. DNA testing methods have enabled microbiologists to identify over five hundred different microorganisms that dwell in the human mouth. In the future, dentists will be able to use DNA testing of your saliva to accurately pinpoint the pathogens causing damage in your mouth and select the proper antibiotics or treatments to eradicate those organisms. Until that time (and even after), the best we can do for our teeth is to brush and floss as often as possible, and see our dentist often for cleaning and maintenance.

12 Hair Today, Hair Tomorrow

Keeping what you've got and growing more

Let me state it flatly, there is no cure for baldness . . . yet. *However, there is much we can do to conserve what we have and much we can do to restore some of what we've lost.* When it comes to hair loss, there are many variables to be considered; what leads to it may be precipitated by different and overlapping events both for men and women (although it is a much more frequent problem in men than in women).

Common hair loss, called androgenetic alopecia (AGA)—also called hereditary hair loss, pattern hair loss, and male pattern baldness—accounts for about 95 percent of all cases of hair loss in the United States. Aging, hereditary factors, stress, illness, any number of medications, surgery, and immune system problems can cause hair loss. Many postmenopausal women experience thinning hair as a result of changing hormones; also pregnancy, nutritional imbalances, chemotherapy, and radiation treatments can cause hair loss.

This chapter will concentrate on hair loss brought on primarily by the processes of aging. AGA occurs as a combination of various dynamics coming together to produce hair loss:

- hormonal changes

- genetic expression

- immunological factors

- oxidative damage

- diminished circulation

To address this problem, there are countless products available, some effective, some not. I've researched the field thoroughly for what I believe to be the most effective measures for keeping what you've got, preventing further loss—perhaps growing some back. But first, let's look at some of the many causes of AGA as we understand them today.

Here's How You Lose Your Hair

The most current scientific theories about balding implicate a major metabolite of the male hormone testosterone called dehydrotestosterone (DHT). This androgen hormone increases as we age when an enzyme called 5-alpha reductase (5AR) reacts with testosterone, converting it to DHT. Our capacity to regulate DHT decreases as we age, enabling it to do all kinds of damage; for instance, it can cause a noncancerous enlargement of the male prostate gland called benign prostate hyperplasia (BPH).

Increased DHT inhibits the growth and shrinks the size of hair follicles. As the hair follicle is affected by DHT, the health and vitality of the surrounding skin also suffer. This stimulates immune system cells to accumulate around the hair follicle, causing damage and inflammation, and at times actually attacking the hair follicle. This sequence of events progressively miniaturizes the involved hair follicle. Over time the smaller follicle goes on to produce a denatured-looking hair, coupled with a shortened growth cycle. So we wind up with peach fuzz for hair, or none at all.

Adding insult to injury, significant changes occur in the structure of the blood vessels leading to the scalp, with a substantial drop-off of the capillaries supplying blood and nutrients to the hair follicle.

A successful treatment protocol has got to utilize a multifaceted approach, bringing together elements that:

- are antiandrogenic, blocking DHT and related androgens

- block free-radical damage at the site

- offer autoimmune protection

- stimulate hair-growth factors

- block any further hair loss

- increase circulation to the follicle and increase hair shaft size

These are tall orders, which can be fulfilled by following the Healthy High-Tech Body recommendations. Of course, if you want to get the best results in hair conservation and restoration, you should be eating well, exercising, and taking appropriate nutraceuticals.

There are several on-line sites that are exceptional if you want to go even further in your search for the ultimate information on hair and to procure some of the products I recommend:

- One of the most comprehensive and well researched is MPB Research; contact them at http://hairloss-research.org.

- Go to www.smart-drugs.net for up-to-the-minute research on hair conservation and for tracking down several great products available only overseas or through mail order at their site.

- Go to Skin Biology at www.folligen.com for amazing research information on hair and the best *copper peptide* products on the market for promoting hair regrowth.

- Go to www.hairsite.com, a division of MediHair, an overseas supplier of some technically well-developed formulas not available in the United States, such as Propecia in a topical form mixed in with minoxidil.

The Products

Here are some of the most advanced products available, how they work, and how best to combine them:

Minoxidil and Pyridine N-Oxides (NANO)

Minoxidil is a product that was originally developed to lower blood pressure. Patients who took it made a remarkable discovery; not only was their blood pressure going down, their hair was growing back as well! Speculation has it that minoxidil works by imitating growth factors that increase blood supply to the hair follicle, preventing it from resting or dying. Minoxidil (sold commercially under the name Rogaine) works best in the 2 to 5 percent range and is available over the counter. It seems to be most effective in the presence of **retinolic acid**, also known as Retin-A, an antiwrinkle skin cream. The combination enhances both the penetration and hair-growth attributes of minoxidil. The Retin-A also appears to promote healthy skin growth and improved circulation. This combination can be compounded by your dermatologist; it is available on-line at www.medihair.com.

One of the world's great authorities on hair loss is Dr. Peter Proctor, a dermatologist based in Houston, Texas. He currently owns the patent on a natural hair regrowth stimulator that works in a manner similar to minoxidil, known as **pyridine**

n-oxides (also known as "natural" minoxidil or NANO). It is available in a product called Dr. Proctor's Advanced Hair Regrowth Formula. Dr. P's NANO formula also contains SODs (see below). I recommend it because it addresses several of the probable causes of hair loss: immune system irregularities, inflammation, and free-radical damage. *This is an absolute must-have in your medicine cabinet.* It's available through the Life Extension Foundation, along with Dr. Proctor's shampoo and conditioners, which are also highly infused with his "natural" minoxidil. Many people who do not respond well to minoxidil find these products effective.

Folligen

This product is made up of copper peptides, which act both as profound anti-inflammatory agents and as antioxidants when applied directly to the scalp. Copper peptides are among the most powerful hair regrowth stimulators available. They are *super oxide dismutases* (SODs), potent free-radical scavengers that play a critical role in countering the excessive free-radical damage that happens throughout the scalp and follicles. The active copper peptides in Folligen have been shown to stimulate skin repair while possessing anti-inflammatory properties.

Folligen is the creation of Dr. Loren Pickheart, whose earlier hair inventions led to the development of **Tricomin**, a commercially available product for stimulating hair growth, and **GraftCyte**, which is used to promote successful grafting in hair transplant surgery. The Folligen products are Dr. Pickheart's latest inventions for hair stimulation. Studies conducted at more than thirty leading universities and medical research institutes led by dermatologists and scientists have thoroughly established the effectiveness of the *copper-peptide technologies* for hair and skin tissue regeneration. *This is undeniably a required product for anyone seriously concerned about hair loss.* It may also be that the SODs inhibit the localized immune response that causes so much hair loss and offset damage and inflammation already incurred. Without dealing with the immunological factors involved in the hair loss process, the potential for hair regrowth is limited.

Propecia

Propecia is used to regrow hair by blocking the action of 5AR, which means that it stops testosterone from becoming DHT. In high doses of up to 5 milligrams, this product is called Proscar and is used to protect the male prostate gland from benign prostate hyperplasia. In low doses of 1 milligram, the product is called Propecia, which studies have shown to be effective for preventing hair loss. It also helps some people regrow hair. The website www.medihair.com offers a version of Propecia formulated with minoxidil in various strengths to apply locally. They offer other novel combinations of minoxidil, including one for women suffering hair loss that is formulated with progesterone.

Nizoral Shampoo

This is an antifungal shampoo, designed to kill the fungi that cause seborrhea (oily scalp) and dandruff. Nizoral contains a chemical called ketoconazole, a plant derivative that may be a "weak" DHT inhibitor. It seems to be relatively fast-acting, showing results within a matter of weeks. It may also reduce inflammation at the hair follicle. Nizoral is available in a 1 percent solution over-the-counter in the United States. It is available overseas, and on-line at www.smart-drugs.net in a 2 percent solution, which is recommended for better results. Use it two or three times a week, followed by a high-quality conditioner.

Dercos

This is a recent product developed by L'Oreal Laboratories in France; it contains a drug called aminexil. Here's how it works: their researchers discovered that whether stress, genetics, or hormonal changes are responsible for hair loss, the problem is always accompanied by *perifollicular fibrosis*. This is a condition that causes the collagen around the root of the hair to become rigid. When this occurs, the collagen tightens, pushing the hair root to the surface of the scalp, which causes hair loss, premature and otherwise. It's possible that this condition may also affect the appearance and rapid disappearance of new hair follicles, as they can't be formed deep in the scalp. *Aminexil has been shown to stop perifollicular fibrosis!* In a yearlong study, 350 men and women who applied Dercos to their scalps for eight weeks showed significantly more hair regrowth than those using a placebo. It's currently available in France and Germany and on-line at www.smart-drugs.net.

In Conclusion: The Healthy High-Tech Body Program for Hair Conservation

The program I propose below is an effective way of addressing your hair loss concerns. It constitutes a "stack," not unlike grouping or stacking supplements to produce a richer, synergistic effect. This then is my basic grouping of products to produce the most measurable results. I recommend that as you become familiar with the products and how they work, you experiment with newer additions, so as to rotate in new ones that may hit some angle possibly missed by the current stack you're using:

Hair Regrowth Program

Basic To-Do

1 Depending on how often you shampoo your hair, use Nizoral shampoo two or three times a week, leaving it on your scalp for five minutes. Rotate with Folligen Therapy Shampoo for the remaining days you wash your hair. Leave it in for five minutes, then rinse. Use either Dr. Proctor's NANO conditioner or the Folligen conditioner.

2 Apply Dr. Proctor's Advanced Hair Regrowth Formula, using eight to ten drops on the thinning areas of your hair. Do this every morning. You can mix this in with minoxidil formulated with Retin-A.

3 Apply Folligen every night before bedtime, in the thinning/balding areas. I recommend that you periodically brush this in, to stimulate it deeper into your scalp. You may also combine it with minoxidil. Apply minoxidil first, let it dry, then apply Folligen over it.

Advanced Protocols

- Use Dercos ampules as directed by the manufacturer.

- Use minoxidil with Retin-A, on a rotation basis.

- Use minoxidil compounded with progesterone (if you're a woman).

- Use Propecia (1 milligram daily).

- Use the amino acid lysine, approximately 500 to 2,000 milligrams a day. In combination with the above protocols involving 5AR inhibitors and minoxidil, lysine is an effective potentiating agent for hair regrowth. An English biotech company (Bio-Scientific Ltd.) was recently issued a U.S. patent for the use of lysine, an amino acid for the treatment of various forms of hair loss, including androgenic alopecia. I would highly recommend using a combination supplement, **Arginine Pyroglutamate with Lysine** by Ultimate Nutrition. You get not only the high dose of lysine but also the growth support factors of several nutrients combined.

What the Future Holds

Dr. Michael Hollick of Boston University Medical Center is developing parathyroid blocking compounds that will work by turning cell division back on, thus stimulating hair regrowth. Anti Cancer Inc. of La Jolla, California, is developing a treatment that will deactivate the baldness gene. It will likely be a topical cream intended to be used daily. A number of companies worldwide are developing varieties of next-generation 5AR inhibitors, which hit both Type I and Type II DHT conversion. One of these drugs, which is being developed by GlaxoSmithKline, is called dutasterida. In clinical trials, it has shown dramatic success in restoring hair for bald men. It is taken in tablet form and works by interferring with the enzymes that break down testosterone and turn it into DHT.

The most powerful DHT blocker yet developed is **RU58841**, made by the Roussel Corporation of France. It produces no systemic side effects whatsoever, leaving the rest of the body completely unaffected. It also appears to induce hair growth for many people who have previously been unsuccessful. However, this is a powerful drug that is still in early test stages and may be for quite some time.

Although we haven't talked about hair transplants in this chapter, there are some new developments on that front as well. Recent experiments have been conducted transplanting hair cells from one individual to another in order to stimulate hair growth in the recipient. In one such experiment, tissue was taken from one researcher and transplanted into another, generating new hair follicles along with new hair in a five-week period. What's amazing is that the recipient did not immunologically reject the tissue. So within the next two decades, you just may be able to have your own hair cloned and "seeded" back into your scalp.

CAN PROTEIN GROW HAIR? A study reported in the February 19, 2001, issue of the *Journal of Clinical Investigation* reported that researchers had discovered a protein normally associated with blood vessel growth that makes hair follicles grow bigger. The protein, called vascular endothelial growth factor (VEGF), is currently used to help heart patients grow blood vessels. Studies were conducted on mice. One group was genetically bred to produce extra VEGF. These mice grew fur faster and thicker than their "normal" counterparts. When hair was shaved off, it grew back 70 percent thicker than normal mouse hair. But don't get too excited just yet. Scientists are now working on a way to get VEGF into the scalp in a cream or ointment, and they have no idea if it will work on humans.

13 High-Level Fitness

Exercising twenty-first-century options

Every few blocks in New York City, you notice a lot of new construction and renovation. And while many of these sites turn into the ubiquitous Starbucks, many others become fitness centers. They're everywhere. You'd think that New York was filled with healthy, buffed bodies. Not so.

Not only is New York short of well-toned residents, so is the rest of the country. Despite the fact that we all know the importance of physical activity, most of us are still couch-bound. According to the Centers for Disease Control and Prevention, half the adults in America are considered overweight and about 18 percent are obese. And yet, the level of physical activity among adults did not change from 1990 to 1998, when only 25 percent of adults (eighteen and over) met basic physical activity recommendations: at least thirty minutes of moderate-intense exercise, such as brisk walking, five days a week, or at least twenty minutes of intense exercise, such as running or aerobics, three days a week.

In fact, it turns out that most people are indifferent when it comes to exercise—thus the high rates of obesity, diabetes, and heart disease.

This indifference could be dangerous for our species.

Stu Mittleman, one of America's most well-known fitness educators and endurance athletes and the author of *Slow Burn,* explains that, once again, we've got to look back to our evolutionary roots to understand what has happened to our bodies. We get energy from two sources: fat and sugar. In general, our bodies rely on fat for the energy we need. In emergency situations, where the fight-or-flight response takes over, we turn to sugar to get us through. "Now, however, because of our sedentary lifestyles, we are not active enough for this fat-based energy system," says Mittleman. "Then when we do exercise, we tend to do too much. We put ourselves into this sugar-burning, anaerobic situation. The end result is that as we burn sugar, which produces acid, we turn into sugar-burning, acid-forming machines. The body then produces cholesterol as a protective device against the corrosive effect of the acid in the tissues. The cholesterol buildup then leads to plaque buildup, which leads to severe disease."

Obviously, not everyone fits into the category of inactive couch potato; those new fitness centers do not go empty. Many of us do take time out of our impossibly busy lives to get in some exercise. And then there are people who take fitness one step beyond, people whose goal is to test the limits of human performance potential. They are looking to go beyond the minimum requirements for health and into the next level of fitness.

Muscles and Genes

You have more muscle tissue in your body than any other kind. Muscle not only enables you to move around but also acts as a storage facility for many of the body's essential substances, such as amino acids—the building blocks of protein. That means that when you lose muscle mass, you also lose protein and weaken your immune system.

There are many different types of muscle in the body, including heart muscle, but skeletal muscle is the most abundant. A muscle is actually a bundle of fibers kept together by collagen tissue. There are two types of muscle fiber, Type I and Type II, also known as slow and fast. Slow fibers are important for activities that require endurance, such as long-distance running, cycling, and swimming. Fast fibers are important in shorter-term activities, such as sprinting and weight lifting. Most people have equal amounts of fast and slow fibers. Some individuals have a higher proportion of one than the other; that's why one person may be better suited as a marathon runner than as a sprinter or vice versa.

In the past two decades, researchers have uncovered some interesting facts about muscle plasticity. It turns out that under various circumstances, muscle fibers can change their size and type. Slow fibers can become fast fibers, and vice versa. It also turns out that there are actually two fast fibers, Type IIx and Type IIa. While Type IIa fibers can sustain an output of power for a longer time period, Type IIx fibers are faster, more powerful, and more quickly fatigued.

When you exercise heavily, as in weight training, Type IIx fibers decrease and Type IIa fibers increase. What happens when you stop exercising? The answer can provide a helpful training tip: it turns out that when the training stops, Type IIx fibers return in even greater numbers than before (although eventually they return to normal levels). So if you are a sprinter facing a major competition, your best training technique would be to train heavily, then give yourself some time off before your race to let the Type IIx fibers build up, and then compete.

Bulking Up with Neutraceuticals

Suppose you're not in training for a particular sport or event, but you exercise regularly and want to pump it up just a little. You might want to consider some of the supplements described in chapter 5 (under the heading "Muscle Building and Power") and add your contribution to the more than $800 million spent on sports supplements each year. Supplements alone cannot make you stronger or give you more endurance. But when coupled with an appropriate fitness routine, they can elevate energy levels and help repair damaged tissue.

Here is a recap of those supplements most helpful in increasing the efficiency of your workouts:

Creatine Monohydrate

Creatine naturally occurs in your body. When you contract your muscle, you break down the chemical *adenosine tri-phosphate* (ATP) into two other chemicals, *adenosine di-phosphate* (ADP) and inorganic phosphate. This process releases the energy that gives your muscles power. Unfortunately, ATP is used up almost instantaneously. Fortunately, your muscles contain creatine phosphate, which is used to replenish ATP. Eventually, however, your supply of creatine phosphate runs down, and so do you. Taking this supplement can increase the amount of creatine phosphate available to your muscles, thereby increasing the amount of energy available, allowing you to exercise with greater intensity and build up your muscles.

HMB

HMB, or *beta-hydroxy beta-methylbutyrate*, is also produced naturally in the body. It is an amino acid that prevents muscle breakdown, boosts strength levels, and increases muscle size. It can also be found in some foods, such as grapefruit and catfish, but it would be difficult to consume enough of these foods to get the benefits of HMB. Scientists are not exactly sure how HMB works, but it appears that it aids in minimizing protein breakdown that can occur after intense exercise. Some studies have even shown that HMB can help in reducing cholesterol levels.

ZMA

ZMA is *zinc monomethionine aspartate.* It is often combined with magnesium aspartate. Its primary goal, like the other products in this category, is to boost strength levels, prevent muscle tissue breakdown, and enhance muscle size and definition. ZMA has also been shown to increase testosterone levels.

OKG

This is a bond of the amino acid *ornithine* and *alpha ketoglutarate*, an "energy cycle" intermediate nutrient found in our bodies. This, along with the other products in this category, offers a wide range of muscle and strength building properties. It also decreases protein breakdown, increases human growth hormone, and promotes fat loss.

Building the High-Tech Muscle

Skeletal muscle tissue is not only abundant but is also one of the most adaptable tissues in the body. Extensive weight training can double or triple the size of a muscle. When you increase the size of a muscle, you are not forming new fibers, you are increasing the thickness of existing fibers. As we age, we naturally lose muscle fibers. We can't get them back once they're gone, but we can continue to build up the fibers that remain.

The high-performance athlete, however, isn't interested in simply maintaining good muscle tone. We know this from every recent Olympic competition. In the 1950s, weight lifters from the Soviet Union began using anabolic steroids, which are synthetic versions of testosterone (which plays an important part in building muscles). The use of anabolic steroids can be extremely dangerous, however. The Steroid Abuse website (www.steroidabuse.org) lists such possible side effects as breast growth in men, balding, acne, shrunken testicles, stunted height, hostility and aggression, heart disease, and prostate, liver, and kidney cancer—among others. Needless to say, these muscle-building substances are now illegal.

That doesn't mean that elite athletes have given up on finding ways to enhance performance. Here are some of the methods that are currently under way or may be coming soon to an athlete near you:

Blood doping Blood doping made news during the 1984 Olympic games when it was used by the U.S. cycling team. This is how it works: first, one or two pints of blood are removed from your system, frozen, and stored. For the next few weeks, your body—specifically your bone marrow—produces more blood cells to replace the ones that were lost. Then, a day or two before you go into competition, the stored blood is returned to your system, creating a surplus of red blood cells. This enables your circulatory system to carry more oxygen, resulting in more efficient muscle performance and greater endurance. The downside is that doping increases the viscosity of the blood (see chapter 7, "The Power Brain"), forcing the heart to work harder, which can have dire consequences.

EPO This is a peptide hormone called *erythropoetin* that is found naturally in the body. A genetically engineered version was created in 1985 to treat anemia in patients with kidney disease. Now, instead of having to transfuse their own red blood cells back into their bodies, athletes can inject EPO, causing the body to make the cells. This, too, is illegal for Olympic athletes. It is difficult to detect because EPO appears naturally in the body, however, officials can test for the percentage of red blood cells. The normal percentage is about 42 to 43 percent; anyone who is found with a percentage higher than 50 is banned from participating.

Human growth hormone This is becoming the hormone of choice for many athletes because it stimulates growth of both bone and muscle. It, too, is difficult to detect because it occurs naturally in the body. So many athletes used hGH, that many participants called the 1996 Atlanta Olympics "the hGH games."

Gene doping We already know that the IGF-1 growth factor plays an important part in increasing muscle mass; the study that injected IGF-1 into a mouse's leg showed an increase of 15 percent—without exercise. It may be that in the near future, genetic manipulation will replace performance-enhancing drugs. Gene doping could be used to transform muscle fiber types into the one most needed by a particular athlete. Or a gene could be encoded for one of the hormones that promotes muscle growth. There are, of course, major kinks still to be worked out in this technique. For example, a gene implanted to signal muscle growth would probably make skeletal muscles larger. But it might also make the heart muscle larger, which could lead to life-threatening complications.

Exercise and Longevity: Lifting Weights, Maintaining Muscle Mass, and More

For years, exercise experts everywhere have been spouting the benefits of aerobics. We've been told that we must get our hearts pumping, get those bodies moving, sweat, sweat, sweat. The benefits of aerobic exercise have been proven over and over again. They are there, they are true, and they are not to be ignored.

However, many experts are now coming to the conclusion that aerobics alone are not enough. If we look at the Paleofitness model of our ancestors, we see that their daily activities—the ones that kept them in shape—consisted of many different kinds of movement. Yes, they hunted game and ran from predators (keeping them aerobically fit), but they also did a lot of lifting and carrying, a natural form of weight training we now do at the gym.

In the past few years, there has been a subtle shift toward recognizing the importance of weight training. Jonny Bowden, fitness guru and author of *Shape Up!*, puts it this way: "You don't want to have to make a choice between aerobics and weight training; they both have benefits. But the fact is when you gain muscle, you become a better calorie burner. Your metabolism is more efficient. If you do nothing but aerobics, you don't gain as much strength. And as time goes on, your body will continue to break down your muscle tissue unless you take steps to preserve it."

Weight training seems to be particularly important as we age. As we get older, we gain body fat and lose muscle; in fact, we lose about a third of a pound of muscle every year after the age of forty. The good news is that it is never too late to add exercise, especially weight training, to your routine. Dr. William Evans, director of the Nutrition, Metabolism, and Exercise Laboratory at the University of Arkansas, conducted studies with adults as old as one hundred years. Putting them on weight-training programs tripled their muscle strength, improved their balance, and increased their overall activity level.

He told the *Washington Post* in April 2000 that his research "demonstrated that the only way to bring back muscle you have lost is by strength training. This involves lifting a weight or using a machine that provides resistance. The weight should 'fatigue' your muscle after only 10 lifts. If you can lift a weight 20 times it is much too light. We have been able to demonstrate that strength training increases muscle mass . . . increases bone density, stimulates how many calories your body burns up every day . . . and has many other important and positive effects."

Some of those positive effects include:

- reduced tendency to lower-back injuries

- reduced frequency of falling

- decrease in risk of adult-onset diabetes

- increase in HDL cholesterol levels

- elevated mood and temperament

The usual method of strength training is to lift a weight for five to seven seconds, then lower it in the same amount of time, and do several repetitions of this movement. Some research has shown, however, that slower may be better. Instead of lifting the weight for seven seconds, you now take as long as fourteen seconds to lift, and ten seconds to bring it down for fewer repetitions—as low as five per set. Results have shown a gain of up to 50 percent more muscle strength in ten weeks.

DON'T GIVE UP THE AEROBICS! There are still plenty of reasons to keep doing aerobics as you age. Here are a few of them:

- *Aerobic activity sets off the release of hGH.* People tend to get sedentary as they get older, when hGH production is in decline. Becoming more active can elevate those hGH levels, helping to increase muscle mass, shed body fat, and instill a new vitality.

- *Regular exercise strengthens the immune system.* A study reported in the December 2000 issue of *Medicine and Science in Sports and Exercise* looked at 112 frail men and women (average age of seventy-nine) and compared the effects of an enriched diet on the immune system against a regular exercise program. The results showed that the enriched diet had no effect on immune response. However, the group that had exercised responded more strongly to pathogens and researchers concluded that exercise may prevent or slow the age-related decline in immune response.

- *Aerobic exercise improves high-level brain function in older people.* A study at Duke University in 1999 involving 156 people between the ages of fifty and seventy-seven showed that aerobic exercise not only lifted depression but also improved patients' memories as well as their abilities to plan, organize, and juggle different intellectual tasks.

- *Exercise (both aerobic and strength training) promotes pleasure pathways.* A study in the February 2001 issue of *The Lancet* revealed that obese people have fewer dopamine receptors in their brains. Dopamine stimulates the brain to produce feelings of pleasure and satisfaction. Their brains are similar to drug addicts' in that respect. Scientists previously thought that drug addicts got more pleasure from drugs than other people. Now they think they get less pleasure, thus they need more drugs to compensate. This study finds that perhaps overeating is the same—obese people need more food than others to feel satisfied. The solution? Exercise. Exercise activates dopamine circuits, making it easier to feel satisfied.

Proponents say this technique works because the slow lifting puts greater demands on the muscle, almost to the point of failure, which induces the body to build more muscle. More muscle burns calories faster, even when at rest. This technique should be practiced no more than twenty minutes at a time and no more than every other day, because the body needs time to repair and rebuild.

The best exercise routine may just turn out to be what is called circuit training—moving back and forth between various types of exercise. So you might do fifteen minutes on the treadmill, alternate it with ten minutes of free weights, move to the bicycle for fifteen minutes, then go back to the free weights for ten minutes. Not only is this type of routine less boring, it can take you to the next level of endurance, strength, and even weight loss.

The Flexibility Factor: Reducing the Wear and Tear

One of the major problems that face the aging population today is arthritis. Since we live so much longer than our ancestors did, we have much more wear and tear on our joints. Most people have some degree of arthritis by the time they're sixty-five years old. It's estimated that by the year 2020, sixty million Americans will suffer from arthritis.

Arthritis is actually a term that refers to more than one hundred disorders that can cause joints to become damaged or inflamed. The most common type is osteoarthritis, in which bones and cartilage deteriorate. The second most common type is rheumatoid arthritis, in which the immune system (for reasons that are still unknown) begins attacking the joints.

As yet, there is no cure for either form of the disease. The first line of defense is, as always, eating a proper diet and keeping physically active. Regular exercise is extremely important because it builds and maintains the muscle strength necessary to support the joints.

Rheumatoid Arthritis

There are several ways to attack this disease in order to reduce pain and inflammation and slow the progress of joint damage. Some of those therapies include:

Nonsteroidal anti-inflammatory drugs (NSAIDs) These include aspirin and ibuprofen.

COX-2 inhibitors COX-2 enzymes cause pain and inflammation. COX-2 inhibitors restrain that enzyme, while ignoring the COX-1 enzyme, which helps protect the lining of the stomach. COX-2 inhibitors have fewer side effects than NSAIDs. There are currently two COX-2 inhibitor drugs for arthritis: Celebrex and Vioxx. A third drug, Mobic, has been used in Europe for several years and has recently received FDA approval.

TNF inhibitors These are some of the newest drugs in the arthritis arsenal. TNF stands for tumor necrosis factor, which is a cytokine. Cytokines regulate the functions of many cells, including those involved in inflammation. People with rheumatoid arthritis have elevated levels of TNF in their bloodstream. A new drug called etanercept, marketed under the names Enbrel and Remicade, binds with the TNF molecule, preventing it from producing inflammation. This drug is still rather expensive and can only be taken in injectable form, but it has proven to be quite effective.

Bromelain An enzyme found in pineapple that has anti-inflammatory properties, Bromelain has long been used as a folk remedy for arthritis, but in 2000, a German company developed a prescription formula called Phlogenzym that has proven to be effective without causing the stomach problems that are a side effect of NSAIDs.

Olive oil A 1999 report published in the *American Journal of Clinical Nutrition* studied people in Greece, where olive oil is an ingredient in almost every dish. The study found that people who consumed the least amount of olive oil had two and a half times the risk of developing rheumatoid arthritis compared with people who consumed the most. Olive oil is rich in oleic acid, which has strong anti-inflammatory properties.

Osteoarthritis

As we get older, the cartilage that covers the ends of the bones begins to wear away. Osteoarthritis usually affects the joints of the knees, back, and fingers. It is a progressive, degenerative disease. There are several therapies that have been found to relieve much of the pain and symptoms of this type of arthritis as well:

Glucosamine sulfate This is a synthetic version of a natural substance essential for manufacturing cartilage. If the production of glucosamine slows down, so does the production of cartilage. Taking glucosamine in supplement form seems to trigger the joint to produce some of its own. It also enhances joint mobility and decreases joint pain. Veterinarians have been using glucosamine since 1992 for race horses, farm animals, and domestic pets. Since then it has proved effective on humans as well. In fact, more arthritics now take glucosamine than take traditional painkillers and NSAIDs. In January 2001, a study appeared in *The Lancet* that showed for the first time that glucosamine sulfate could actually slow the progression of osteoarthritis. Patients who took glucosamine sulfate tablets for three years showed significant improvement in pain and disability, whereas patients who took a placebo for the same amount of time worsened.

Chondroitin Often taken in combination with glucosamine, chondroitin is made of a complex group of sugar molecules categorized as glycosaminoglycans, which is the main ingredient of cartilage. Chondroitin helps to reform damaged cartilage and to reduce inflammatory conditions. Chondroitin sulfate has been known to lower cholesterol, reduce blood clots, inhibit plaque formation, and improve circulation.

MSM or methylsulfonylmethane This is a form of sulfur that is found naturally in fresh fruits, vegetables, and many other foods. Sulfur is a fundamental building material of our bodies and is essential to our survival. Sulfur is used by the body to form crucial proteins and amino acids. MSM has an incredibly wide array of benefits, including reduced joint pain and stiffness and reduced inflammation.

It really doesn't matter whether you are an elite athlete, a weekend warrior, or a mall walker. What does matter is that you start right now to consider the benefits of exercise—High Tech or otherwise. Physical activity seems to be a requirement of retaining quality of age into our twilight years (however old that may turn out to be).

Pillar 5

Sexuality

In his movie *Sleeper*, Woody Allen envisioned the Orgasmatron.

In his twenty-first century, you needed a machine to enhance your sexuality. In our twenty-first century, you are the machine programmed to enhance your own sexuality.

Whatever your age, whichever your gender, you are a sexual creature. Every animal is, and we are no different. In chapter 14, simply called "Sex," you'll discover exactly what you need to know to retain a healthy, vibrant sexuality throughout your life, even into old age. I'll tell you what science knows—and what it doesn't—about the things that happen to our reproductive systems as we age.

I'll tell you about "male menopause" and what you should do about it. I'll talk about PMS and female menopause, and how to treat them. I'll clue you in on the latest drugs and hormone replacement therapies for both men and women, and why you should or should not consider them. Advancing age is not a reason to give up on sexuality. With a Healthy High-Tech Body, you can hang a sign on your door at any age that says, "No Orgasmatron needed here!"

14 Sex

Solutions to sexual perplexities

Sex. Sexuality. This is way too big a topic for me to give it the full Healthy High-Tech Body treatment I'd prefer to at least in this book—*sex*, that is. There are academic volumes and institutions in this field that cover and have covered the subject matter in ways I can't begin to approach here; it simply isn't within the capacity or the mission of *The Healthy High-Tech Body*. I'm hardly an expert on human sexuality, but I'm a participant and a fan of it, with an innate interest and fascination with the subject matter.

This chapter isn't a primer on relationships or marriage. It's not intended to provide the keys to any of the nuances, subtleties, mystery, chemistry, magic, and ritual of human sexuality.

It is, however, a guide to enhancing your sexual experience, especially if you're having problems in that area, whether you're a man or a woman. The recommendations in this chapter are designed to help you maintain and enhance sexual performance, and to enjoy sex throughout your life. I do not promise you the degree of sexual performance you may have experienced or exhibited in high school or college. This is a complex, sometimes confusing subject. This chapter will present you with what science currently knows, and with what High-Tech doctors and pharmacologists are doing to help create a healthier sexuality that does not have to diminish as we age.

Where Do We Begin?

If you want to maintain a healthy, active sexuality throughout your life (and who doesn't?), you will have to approach the situation from a variety of angles. You'll have to use a *multimodal strategy* along a number of parameters affecting sexual expression.

There are hormonal issues to contend with, for both men and women. Hormones alter as we age, affecting our sex drive. (This term has come to encompass the full expression of sexuality, including the interest generated by the brain, which is a primary sexual organ, the central nervous system, and the actual performance of your sex organs.)

There are health and fitness issues, which were covered in earlier sections of this book, that play central roles in the experience of sex. Your stress hormones, for instance, affect your sex hormones. Too much stress and you impair sexual performance. If you have high blood viscosity as an effect of elevated blood lipid levels, circulation will be impaired to your sex organs, affecting everything from signals from the brain all the way down to blood flow directly into the penis or clitoris. The sexual experience is "global"; that is to say it happens all over our bodies in a full sensorial cascade of feelings. Even these sensations of pleasure can be dampened in a less than fit body. So you can see that staying fit throughout your life is a central part of the *multimodal approach* to enhanced sexual drive.

Andropause: Hormone Changes and the Male Menopause

In most regards, it is easier to target the problems of male sexual performance, given the obvious differences between male and female sex organs. One of the biggest problems for men over forty is the change in testosterone, the primary male hormone, in particular the levels of *free testosterone* circulating in the blood. This decline is called *andropause*, and is sometimes referred to as the male menopause. According to Dr. Jeremy Heaton, head of urology at Queen's University in Ontario, "There is no such thing as male menopause—if you underline the pause. It's not like women who stop menstruating. Men do not stop functioning. But there is definitely a syndrome where a number of different bodily functions slow down and really begin to affect men from a clinical, everyday-life standpoint."

Here's a quick run-through of what happens: as men age, declining levels of testosterone (testosterone deficit) begin to contribute to abdominal weight gain, depression, elevated cholesterol, and other conditions associated with aging. In his book *The Testosterone Syndrome,* Dr. Eugene Shippen argues that a range of testosterone deficit–induced problems can be seen in a multitude of health conditions in the aging male: "The changes seen in aging, such as the loss of lean body mass, the decline in energy, strength and stamina, unexplained depression and decrease in sexual sensation and performance are all directly related to testosterone deficiency. Degenerative diseases such as heart disease, stroke, diabetes, arthritis, osteoporosis, and hypertension are all linked directly or indirectly to testosterone decline. . . ."

Part of this aging is a kind of "feminizing effect" as male estrogen levels (you read right) begin to increase as part of the aging process itself, blocking the ability of testosterone to work effectively in the brain, nerves, muscles, and genitals. It is important to keep testosterone in the *free* form in our bloodstream to "activate" the proper cell receptors involved in our libido.

If you are a male with diminished sex drive, the first thing to do is to get tested. You need the proper bloodwork to determine if low levels of both *free* and *total testosterone* are at the root of your problem (see chapter 10 on diagnostics for the proper tests to request). It's a well-documented fact that middle-aged men with testosterone deficit often have difficulty getting aroused and/or staying aroused long enough to enjoy having sex. Sexual arousal begins in your brain, with neuronal testosterone receptors stimulated by the presence of the hormone. If there are inadequate amounts of testosterone present, arousal will not occur.

Once you've determined that your hormone levels are low, there are a number of ways to normalize them, to bring them back to acceptable levels. There are several excellent books that go into great detail on the subject that I recommend you read before discussing your options with your doctor:

- *Maximize Your Vitality and Potency* by Dr. Jonathan Wright

- *The Testosterone Syndrome* by Dr. Eugene Shippen, M.D.

- *Super T* by Dr. Carliss Uliss

- "Male Hormone Modulation Therapy" section, on-line at www.oz.lef.org.

It is possible to use synthetic testosterone prescribed by your doctor. A better plan of action might be to use natural testosterone such as **androderm**, which is available in patch form and is FDA-approved for men with insufficient levels of testosterone.

A second line of support is to use a *nutraceutical* that contains dietary nutrients known to block undesirable levels of estrogen in men and increase levels of desirable free testosterone:

C h r y s i n   This is a plant extract known as a bioflavionoid that blocks aromatase, the enzyme that triggers testosterone conversion into estrogen. The less testosterone that is converted, the more there is available to you. Chrysin is added to many products used by bodybuilders as part of their muscle-fitness programs. It is also a potent antioxidant and has been shown to reduce inflammation. It may also play a role in moderating the undesirable effects of stress hormones in our body. It appears that this plant compound works best in the presence of piperine (an extract of pepper) or other plant-based bioflavionoids.

I recommend a nutraceutical formula by the Life Extension Foundation called MiraForte with Chrysin. LEF has conducted extensive studies on their formulation, which includes a number of additional herbs like nettle root extract and muira puama.

Nettles Nettles work by inhibiting the form of testosterone known as DHT in the blood, which can lead to premature hair loss and to prostate enlargement. It also controls the levels of sex hormone binding globulin (SHBG), which renders free testosterone inactive—something we don't want to happen.

Muira Muira is a libido enhancer that comes from the stems and roots of a plant found in the Amazon region of South America. It has been the subject of two published clinical studies conducted by Dr. Jacques Waynberg of the Institute of Sexology in Paris, France, and reported as far back as 1994 in the *American Journal of Natural Medicine*. The studies outline the broad impact that muira has on a range of parameters affecting sexual function, including the inability to maintain an erection. It is presently being marketed as a natural Viagra by various manufacturers. Muira probably works by favorably altering the hormone balance in the aging male. It also seems to reverse much of the physical discomfort associated with lower levels of testosterone, including fatigue and loss of strength.

The Future of Sexual Performance: Beyond Viagra

Scientists are currently working on several drugs and combinations of drugs that work in the brain and also produce the best local effect—a cocktail of sorts that would affect the pleasure centers in the brain and increase localized sensation in the genital area. Let's look at what's coming up:

Viagra

It's hard to imagine anyone on the planet who hasn't heard of Viagra. Annoying as those "celebrity" endorsements are (you know who you are, Bob Dole), they have served to raise awareness of the problem of erectile dysfunction. Many men who were previously embarrassed to bring up the subject with their doctors are suddenly eager to ask for Viagra. In fact, in the few years since Pfizer introduced this drug, it has become one of the biggest-selling drugs in history with more than twenty million prescriptions to date.

Viagra increases a naturally produced enzyme called cyclic GMP (guanosine monophosphate) that is essential to maintain an erection and blocks an enzyme known as phosphodiesterase Type 5 (PDE-5). Doing so increases blood flow to the penis, resulting in improved erections and rigidity. It also increases genital sensitivity in women. It doesn't work on increasing your *desire or appetite* for sex; it does, however, increase sensation on a local level. Viagra does have side effects. Some patients have reported congestion, diarrhea, facial flushing, and headaches. A small percentage of men also report temporary changes in visual acuity, including light sensitivity and a bluish tinge to their vision. And men who suffer from heart disease, especially those who take nitroglycerin medication, are advised never to take Viagra.

VIAGRA FOR WOMEN? It seems that Viagra is not just for men anymore. A study conducted out of Boston University Medical Center evaluated thirty-five women, mean age of fifty, all of whom had hysterectomies. Patients in the study filled out the Brief Index of Sexual Function for Women (BISF-Q) before using Viagra (sildenafil), and then again six weeks after. Before Viagra, all the patients reported low sensation and inability to reach orgasm, and 68 percent reported pain and discomfort. After using Viagra, only 22 percent reported low sensation, only 18 percent reported an inability to reach orgasm, and only 33 percent reported pain or discomfort. The lead doctor of the study, Dr. Jennifer Berman, stated in typical doctorese, "The trends seen here indicate that post-sildenafil hysterectomy patients do experience a statistically significant decrease in symptoms of low sensation."

Alpha MSH or PT-141

This prosexual drug, originally called Melanotan, comes out of the University of Arizona. It was intended to produce a nice tan and help reduce skin cancer. It does produce a beautiful tan; it also produces spontaneous erections. It has a very high success rate and appears to affect both desire and physical performance. Researchers believe the drug acts specifically on a part of the brain known as the hypothalamus, setting off the arousal centers there. It's currently in trials by Palatin Technologies Inc., in both nasal spray and pill form. PT-141 will be useful for both men and women.

Alprostadil

Commercially known as Caverjet, this drug, a prostaglandin preparation, is directly injected into the penis. It works by relaxing the smooth muscle of the penis and the muscles surrounding the arteries, allowing for an increase in blood flow through the *cavernosal* arteries, engorging them and creating an erection. A study published in the March 2001 issue of *Urology* showed that 85 percent of seventy men with erectile dysfunction who used Caverjet over a twelve-month period showed a return of spontaneous erections. Topiglan, a topical gel version of this product (and probably the one most men would prefer) is currently in trials by the MacroChem Corporation.

Apomorphine or Uprima

Uprima was initially investigated as a possible Parkinson's drug. Unlike Viagra, which acts directly on blood flow to the penis, Uprima sparks an erection by stimulating a brain chemical involved in arousal. This is a drug that may work well for people with compromised health issues such as high blood pressure or diabetes who are facing significant levels of erectile dysfunction. It's an option also for men with heart disease who can't use Viagra. There are several studies that have been done on this medication showing just how it works, according to Dr. Jeremy Heaton of Queen's University, who is my favorite researcher in the field of sexual performance. According to Dr. Heaton, Uprima works in the part of the brain where the neurosignaling takes place. The drug assists the brain in converting the desire to have an erection into the actual mechanisms involved in the process. It's extremely fast-acting—ten minutes as opposed to Viagra's one hour. Currently in drug-approval hell, Uprima is made by TAP Holdings.

Verdenafil

This is Bayer's foray into the prosexual drug market. It works similarly to Viagra by inhibiting PDE-5. It may have a slight edge on Viagra in that the studies indicate more men using this drug were able to complete sexual intercourse all the way to ejaculation. It seems to be somewhat more selective than Viagra at targeting the PDE-5 enzyme and works better at lower doses. Awaiting FDA approval, look for it in late 2002.

So for Men . . .

There are a number of other drug candidates in various stages of development. There's one called TA1790, which is supposed to be an even faster-acting, more potent PDE-5 inhibitor, that should be available soon. All of these products come with warnings. Side effects can vary, from nausea to skin flushing to more severe complications, and only you can judge if the end result is worth it. All these medications are or will be available through your doctor or local urologist; all your options should be discussed with your doctor as well as with your significant other.

I've covered most of what's new in male sexual potency and enhancement medication; however, as Dr. Jeremy Heaton told *Men's Journal* in October 2000, "In five to ten years, we'll have a dozen major male prescriptive sex pills, creams, and lozenges on the market, each working a slightly different angle, available to be used separately or in combination by bored adventurers and stressed overachievers to tweak their performance."

Women's Sexuality: Pleasure, Perimenopause, and Menopause

When men have a sexual "problem," it's pretty obvious. They can't get it up. Or they can't keep it up. Or they can get it partway up, but not as up as they'd like it to be. But what about women? Don't they have sexual "problems" as well? Of course they do, even if those same drug companies that are racing to develop products for men have been ignoring that fact for decades. Part of the reason is that female sexual arousal is a much more complex—and in many ways more subtle—subject. Very little is known about how a woman's libido actually functions.

Things are beginning to change. In some ways, women have Viagra to thank for that. When erectile dysfunction came out of the closet, so to speak, women began to talk about their problems as well. And some people began paying attention.

Doctors began listening to women who came in to complain about lack of libido and/or about sexual discomfort, and they began to test these women for low testosterone levels. Many women were found to have subnormal levels. The standard treatment is to take DHEA, which breaks down into usable testosterone. This works for many women. However, testosterone can have unwanted side effects. Too high a dosage can result in deepening of the voice, excessive hair growth, and enlargement of the clitoris.

So other doctors, including Dr. Jed Kaminetsky, a New York urologist, began to look for new solutions. "I have a large practice in male sexual dysfunction," says Kaminetsky. "But it became apparent early on that we were only treating half the problem. We could help men get erections, but it didn't help their sex lives unless their partners were satisfied as well."

Kaminetsky experimented with a variety of substances—some worked but were awkward to use or had annoying side effects. Then when Viagra came out, he found that many women did well on the drug—but many suffered headaches (for real), nausea, congestion, and vision problems. So he started prescribing a topical form of Viagra, which works very well without the side effects.

However, Viagra requires a doctor visit and a prescription. Dr. Kaminetsky wanted to find something that would be available to women everywhere. He began experimenting again, this time focusing on L-arginine, an essential amino acid, one of the building blocks of protein in the body. L-arginine, it turns out, is a precursor to nitric oxide, a potent blood vessel dilator. That means it enlarges the blood vessels in the clitoris, which in turn increases sensitivity. Dr. Kaminetsky developed an L-arginine-based topical cream (you apply it before sex right where it counts) that he calls **Dream Cream**, a nonprescription product that has worked for hundreds of his patients. The result for most women is better lubrication and more arousal and pleasure. And other than a slight warm and/or tingly feeling, it has produced virtually no side effects. (See the resource guide for his address and website.)

So, while Dr. Jeremy Heaton predicts that we'll have dozens of "solutions" for men on the market in the next five years, there's no telling what will be available for women. But it seems as if we may be on the right track.

Perimenopause and Menopause: Sexuality Continues

Perimenopause and menopause are stages in a lengthy process called the *climacteric*, which can begin for women at about age thirty-five and end as late as age sixty. The average age at which American women experience menopause is fifty-one.

The climacteric refers to the hormonal changes that start occurring in women's bodies during these years. Specifically, the ovaries dramatically decrease their production of the female hormones *estrogen* and *progesterone*. Menopause occurs when the ovaries are no longer producing these hormones and the menstrual cycle has ended. Perimenopause begins when these hormone-related changes begin to take place, as long as ten years before menopause. Perimenopause often arrives with varying degrees of discomfort, such as hot flashes, vaginal dryness, mood swings, and often a lowered sex drive. These symptoms are not universal. Some women will experience all of them, some will have no symptoms, and most women will fall somewhere in the middle.

By the year 2020, there will be fifty million women over the age of fifty in America, all of whom will be facing the "problem" of menopause. These fifty million women will probably live longer than most of their ancestors did, and many of them will live a third of their lives after menopause. It's no wonder that it has become such a well-studied topic in recent years.

In fact, the literature on how to address menopause is exhaustive—and confusing. There isn't as direct a way of dealing with the personal events of menopause as there is for the male andropause. Up until recently, the only solution for women was estrogen replacement therapy (ERT), with its heavy-handed use of synthetic estrogen and progesterone.

That is no longer the case. There are new and exciting developments on the horizon. The rest of this chapter will take a look at synthetic hormones and their alternatives. There are important decisions to be made; you may have to try several pathways before you find the right one. And you will have to find a willing and knowledgeable physician to help you make these decisions.

It's important here to note that menopause has been largely *pathologized* in our culture, viewed as an illness to be dealt with as a medical problem requiring intervention and pharmaceutical treatment. A quick look at some facts:

- 46 percent of postmenopausal women in America take or have taken medically prescribed hormone therapy.

- 30 percent of postmenopausal women in Britain and Scandinavia take or have used medically prescribed hormones.

- Continental European use hovers in the lower teens.

- Japanese women come in at a mere 6 percent.

- American women using hormones are likely to have more formal education; by contrast, in Norway the more educated the woman is, the less likely she is to use hormones.

If you are experiencing perimenopause or menopause, your first order of business is to get as much information as possible. I recommend that you read:

- *Before the Change: Taking Charge of Your Perimenopause* by Ann Louise Gittleman

- *Super Nutrition for Menopause* by Ann Louise Gittleman

- *Woman: An Intimate Geography* by Natalie Angier

- *Wisdom of Menopause: Creating Physical and Emotional Well-being During the Change* by Dr. Christiane Northrup

- *Health Wisdom for Women,* newsletter by Dr. Christiane Northrup

- *Fight Fat After Forty* by Dr. Pamela Peeke

- *Natural Hormone Replacement Therapy* by Dr. Jonathan Wright

I also recommend that you visit the following websites:

- www.athena.athene.net

- www.menopause-online.com

- www.wometlc.com

- www.oz.lef.org

Most important, you have to take responsibility for your health, especially where this issue is concerned. The drug companies have a lot at stake in trying to convince you that HRT is the way to go. It may be the appropriate way to go for you. But it behooves you to explore all your options before you make that decision.

The Problems with Synthetic Hormones: Premarin and Provera

One of the most problematic aspects of addressing menopause is that physicians have tended to take a "one size fits all" approach, prescribing the same medications for all women. However, studies have shown that approximately 100,000 women *stop* using HRT because of current and potential side effects. Since these medications are relatively new, the results of long-term studies are just being published.

The synthetic versions of estrogen and progesterone commonly prescribed seem to come with a whole host of side effects and risks, especially the longer they're used. Synthetic estrogen is called Premarin, synthetic progesterone is called Provera, and the combination of both is called Prempro. Provera alone has been shown to decrease blood flow to the heart and the brain, reducing its beneficial effects. A four-year study conducted by Johns Hopkins Medical Center and eighteen other medical centers around the country involving more than 2,700 women concluded—to the surprise of all involved—that "there was no beneficial effect to the hormone therapy," according to Johns Hopkins cardiologist and principal investigator Dr. Roger Blumenthal. He continues, "What is very interesting is that within the first year of the trial there seemed to be an adverse effect of the hormones."

In other words the hormone therapy appeared to raise the risk of a heart attack in the first year, decreasing by year four and leaving no overall benefit. In addition, there was a threefold increase in thromboembolic events (blood clots in the legs and lungs) and a significant increase in gallbladder disease in the user group. In 1995, Graham Colditz and colleagues at the Harvard Medical School followed the health of 122,000 women involved in the Nurses Health Study since 1976. The study results, published in the *New England Journal of Medicine,* claimed that women on HRT therapy had 30 to 40 percent more breast cancer than women who never took hormones. Women aged sixty to sixty-four on HRT for at least five years increased their risk of getting breast cancer by 71 percent and increased their risk of dying from it by 45 percent.

I say let's look at other options.

The Healthy High-Tech Body Program for Hormone Balancing in Women

Test Your Hormones

Although there are a number of medical options for testing for hormones, such as blood and urine sampling, I recommend the use of saliva testing.

Although saliva testing is relatively new to clinical practice, it has more than ten years of research to back it up. It is also supported by a large number of health researchers and practitioners in the field of women's health, including Dr. Christiane Northrup and Ann Louise Gittleman. Saliva collection kits are available through some doctors' offices (those who are familiar with this testing protocol). Saliva test kits can be also be requested directly from two separate laboratories that will provide you with complete kits and prepaid mailers. They are:

- Uni Key Health Systems Inc. (800-888-4353)

- Aeron Lifecycle Clinical Laboratories (800-631-7900)

Both these laboratories will give you and your doctor the proper recommendations for natural hormone replacement therapy. The products these labs recommend are yam or soy based. This technique is also called bioidentical hormone therapy, because it matches female hormones exactly, unlike the synthetics Provera and Premarin.

Natural or Bioidentical Hormone Options

While visiting Clinique La Prairie in Switzerland, I spent time with their resident endocrinologist, hormone, and menopause specialist, Dr. Thierry Pache Appage. Among the things we discussed were the various ways the clinic's doctors approached HRT and their reluctance to use too many hormones to treat menopause. In fact, if anything were needed at all, they might recommend some natural progesterone cream for two weeks out of the month. In case estrogen was required to combat vaginal dryness, Dr. Appage recommended the use of estriol for both perimenopausal and menopausal women. This form of estrogen offers all the benefits of more traditional ERT, without the long-term dangers or side effects.

Back in the States, I had lengthy conversations with Dr. Pamela Peeke, author of *Fight Fat After Forty,* and Ann Louise Gittleman, author of *Before the Change.* They convinced me that many women could manage their hormonal imbalances by using a more moderate approach, using milder products such as estriol and natural progesterone.

As progesterone declines, many women experience a parallel decline in mental clarity, described by a friend of mine as "mental fog." In her case, it did not clear until she started using bioidentical progesterone.

Progesterone has many beneficial properties. It activates cancer-killing cells in the body and reduces the production of a cancer-causing form of estrogen in the blood called 4-hydroxy estrone. It also helps keep up the levels of the good form, estriol. Progesterone has also been shown to increase neuronal energy production and protect brain cells. Progesterone helps to prevent osteoporosis, depression, and a myriad of symptoms harking all the way back to PMS. The best bioidentical progesterone is made from an extract of wild yam called diosgenin. It has to be compounded to look identical to the human progesterone molecule. The product I primarily recommend is **Progesta Key Cream,** by Uni Key Health Systems.

For many women, the use of natural estriol and progesterone may be sufficient. For some women, using naturally compounded testosterone may also make a huge difference in their sense of well-being and their sexual drive. Several different studies have shown conclusively that perimenopausal women with low testosterone levels who exhibited impaired sexual function had greater increases in sexual activity and pleasurable orgasms with the introduction of therapeutic testosterone.

In Conclusion

Going through the climacteric is a personal journey. There are many lifestyle options that will make this journey more pleasant. Diet and exercise, sleep, and stress control all play an important part in the manner in which you navigate this stage of your life. Handled properly, menopause can turn out to be the most extraordinary third of your life.

The 90-Day Healthy High-Tech Body Program

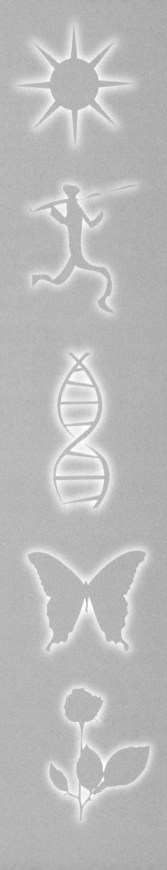

So. You've read the book. If you haven't already, it's time to get started on your way to having a Healthy High-Tech Body. To help you along, I've charted out a 90-day program for you to follow, divided into each of the five pillars.

It's best to start slowly. Follow the suggestions in the chart for the first 30 days. Start by improving your eating habits and getting some exercise. Add in the basics of supplements and detoxification. Get your support systems—your healthcare practitioners and fitness trainers—in place. Begin exploring your options in all categories.

Pick up the pace in the second 30 days. Add more healthy foods and eliminate more toxins. Shed bad habits. You'll begin to feel better and better and, as you move into the third 30 days, you'll be getting the full benefits of the Healthy High-Tech Body program.

Yes, there is work involved. It's not always easy to do what's best for you. You have to remain vigilant, but you don't have to demand perfection. You might even enjoy yourself!

So go to it, and here's to a great ninety years!

First 30 Days

PILLAR 1 Frontiers	PILLAR 2 Supernutrition	PILLAR 3 Life Extension, Life Enhancement	PILLAR 4 The Body Beautiful	PILLAR 5 Sexuality

Consider purchasing at-home diagnostic tools	Follow the Paleotech Diet:
	
	  Add extra servings of fruits and veggies
	
	  Choose lean proteins
	
	  Add fish
	
	Choose menus from Paleotech Gourmet for breakfast, lunch, and dinner
	
	For weight control:
	
	  Eliminate nufoods
	
	  Begin exercise program
	
	  Add fat-burning nutraceuticals
	
	Add supplements from "basics" category
	
	Start basic detox:
	
	  Sauna 15 minutes/ 3 times per week
		Follow steps 1 to 7 of Power Brain preservation
		
		Have all basic diagnostic tests appropriate to your age
		
		Discuss Healthy High-Tech Body with your doctor
		
		Look for Functional Medicine practitioner
		
		Visit your dentist to have teeth checked and cleaned
			Follow ground rules 1 to 4 for great skin and hair
			
			If desired, start preliminary investigation of Botox or laser surgery
			
			Begin basic program with hair conservation products
			
			Institute basic weight-training program
				Evaluate your sexual functioning
				
				Discuss any problems/dissatisfaction/discomfort with your urologist or gynecologist

Second 30 Days

PILLAR 1 Frontiers	PILLAR 2 Supernutrition	PILLAR 3 Life Extension, Life Enhancement	PILLAR 4 The Body Beautiful	PILLAR 5 Sexuality
Sign an organ donor card	Follow the Paleotech Diet: Choose carbs from approved list on glycemic index Reduce consumption of sugar and processed carbs Limit caffeine intake Vary menus from Paleotech Gourmet For weight control: Add second line of fat-burning nutraceuticals Hire personal trainer or join health club Follow Fat Flush Add longer saunas at least twice a month, ½ to 1 hour (in 20-minute increments)	Consider using nootropics Have 6 functional assessments done to cover major body functions	Begin to replace commercial cosmetics with cosmeceuticals If desired, speak with your doctor about Botox or laser surgery Stay vigilant about dental care—brush, floss, and use rubber tip daily Follow High-Tech Body program for hair conservation Consider nutraceuticals to enhance workout efficiency Increase weight-training program If necessary, choose supplements to protect against arthritis	If you have not done so, have hormones checked Discuss options with your healthcare provider; consider natural and bio-identical products

Third 30 Days

PILLAR 1 Frontiers	PILLAR 2 Supernutrition	PILLAR 3 Life Extension, Life Enhancement	PILLAR 4 The Body Beautiful	PILLAR 5 Sexuality

Consider genetic testing if you are at high risk for rare diseases	Continue Paleotech Diet
	
	For weight control:
	
	    Add third line of support products
	
	    Check with physician re possibility/ necessity prescription medication
	
	Add supplements to address your individual problems or concerns (brain performance, muscle enhancement, et cetera)
	
	Visit spa for a supervised power sauna
	
	    Add niacin tweak to sauna
	
	    Add stress management, like massage or yoga
		Continue steps 1 to 7 of Power Brain preservation
		
		If you're considering aggressive approach to anti-aging, investigate injectables, European cell treatments, hGH
		
		Have functional assessments on specific problems or concerns
		
		Consider High-Tech scanning devices for "wellness" diagnostics
			Visit dermatologist for full skin cancer exam
			
			Gradually increase exercise program— aerobics and strength training
				Evaluate use of appropriate products; discuss results and/or side effects with healthcare provider

Epilogue

The problem with doing a book about the future is that the future is always one step ahead of you. It was extremely difficult to finish this book; every day something else would appear in the news that seemed it just had to be included here. Much as I wanted to, I couldn't cover everything. There were many topics I barely touched upon that I would have liked to have presented in depth: cancer, immunology, breakthroughs in psychology. There is just so much to say, so much promise in our High-Tech future—it just wasn't possible to cover it all.

So here's the analogy: you're in the bottom of the third at the World Series. You're in the game. If you follow the rules and play to the best of your potential, you'll keep playing until the ninth inning—maybe longer. Along the way, your pitching arm will probably give out, but modern miracles of sports therapy and bio-mechanics will have you back on the mound in no time. You'll certainly strike out a few times, but you will also hit some incredible homers. But if you take care of yourself along the way, you'll not only get to the end of the game, you'll win the series after all.

That's what it's like to go after a Healthy High-Tech Body. Your goal is to stay in the game as long as possible, playing at peak performance.

It should be clear to you by this point that I'm no Ponce de León searching after the Fountain of Youth. I am after living the best life I possibly can, and helping you to do the same. You get out of the Healthy High-Tech Body what you put into it. You eat better, you feel better. You work out more often, you feel better. You use better nutraceuticals, you feel better. You use better cosmeceuticals, you look better. I know that reading this book isn't going to make you change overnight. My hope is that it will inspire you to change small things all along the way until they build up into the complete Healthy High-Tech you.

The Healthy High-Tech Body can give you unparalleled freedom. If you follow the Healthy High-Tech Body protocols, you can eliminate the boundaries nature imposes on us as we age. You can reduce the limits we put on ourselves by poor nutrition and lack of exercise, by the lack of resources and information. *The Healthy High-Tech Body* has laid it all out for you. Now it's your turn to go after the brass ring. It's definitely within your grasp.

Please, let me know how you're doing. Tell me what has worked for you, and why. Ask me questions. I'll do my best to answer. You can contact me at:

Oz Garcia
10 West 74th Street
New York, NY 10023
info@ozgarcia.com

Or you can always reach me at www.ozgarcia.com. I look forward to hearing from you.

Appendix A: Some Cool Stuff

Appliances for health, comfort, and safety

For many people, the year 1965 has no particular significance. It does for me, however. For me, 1965 was the year I saw the future. It was the year the World's Fair came to New York. I vividly remember riding the subway from the Upper West Side of Manhattan into Queens no less than ten times to visit my favorite pavilion, sponsored by General Motors.

What an incredible future we were to have. There were going to be commuter spaceships shuttling us back and forth to vacation and industrial sites on the moon. Once there, we would ride around in "lunar crawlers." If the moon didn't suit us, we could use our "aqua-scooters" to dive deep underwater to the suboceanic vacation resorts.

Most amazing of all was the city of the future, made up of superskyscrapers, hundreds of stories high. Your hover cars could get you around the city, unless you chose to use the high-speed trains or moving sidewalks. There wasn't much street-level vehicle traffic, because there were underground conveyor belts to deliver the freight.

In the future, we were told, we would live in a leisure society with a three- or four-day workweek. We'd get to work later and leave earlier, and we'd fly off for the long weekends to our country homes, where dinners cooked themselves and robots did the housework.

I was fourteen, and I was enthusiastic and optimistic. I ached to live in such a world.

Fast-forward almost forty years. Is it the future yet? It's certainly not the one I ached to see. I don't know about you, but I'm still searching for that leisure society.

Most of the things in the GM Pavilion did not come to be, and there are so many more things that those GM futurists could never have predicted. As it turns out, the future isn't all that we thought it would be, and the promise of a more comfortable world as a result of technology is a double-edged sword. Technology has made life easier in so many ways—and may be destroying our environment before we all have the time to enjoy it.

There are thousands and thousands of products available to us today to help make us healthier and safer, and to save us from the effects of many of the products we already have. In fact, there are so many it would be impossible to include even a smattering of them here. So I've chosen to highlight ten products, just to give you an idea of what's out there. I'm not endorsing any particular brand of products; I don't have any financial interest in any of them. I'm simply giving you examples from categories of products you might want to explore for your own use.

If you are interested in a particular type of product, comparison shop. Go on the Internet. Get the catalogs. Some of the things you'll find are very strange and of dubious usefulness. But there are many other gadgets, gizmos, and pieces of equipment that really can help your High-Tech Body live in a High-Tech world.

Cool Stuff for Your Personal Health

The Bowflex

Five years ago, realizing that I had less and less time to get to the gym, I started to look for some kind of home fitness equipment that would be sturdy, reliable, and, of course, effective. After several months of research, I discovered the Bowflex. It is basically a strength-training machine, which means that you're doing exercise with resistance. It works your muscles through an entire range of motion, so you get muscle strength instead of muscle bulk.

Instead of piling up weights one on top of the other and then trying to lift them, the Bowflex works via a system of Power Rods. The rods give you the same resistance as the weights, but without the danger or joint pain often associated with free weights. The rods are made of a High-Tech composite material called poly-hexamethaline-adipamide and are guaranteed for life. There are several models of the Bowflex, including one that I particularly admire called the Versatrainer. It is designed specifically for people with limited mobility and disabilities. This is the first piece of home fitness equipment I've found that made these kinds of accommodations. I have to say that, although I'm a three-time marathon veteran, a health and wellness consultant for Equinox fitness clubs, and fitness consultant to the East Coast Alliance of Trainers, over the past five years, my Bowflex has made a real difference in how I look and feel.

You can get more information at www.bowflex.com, or by calling 800-618-8853.

Inversion Therapy

By inverting your body—hanging upside down—your weight provides gentle traction to your spine, expanding the space between the vertebrae and relieving pressure. It can help relieve back pain and spasm caused by compression of the vertebrae—the result of downward loads on muscles, joints, and spine by physical activities such as aerobics, weight lifting, and jogging. It also improves circulation and reduces some of the effects of aging caused by gravity. Inversion tables allow you to lie down and gently rotate through a variety of angles by simple arm movements. The table is equipped with ankle clamps so that you don't slide off. You can find inversion tables in most places that sell fitness equipment, as well as the TechnoScout catalog (800-704-1210), www.technoscout.com, or www.comforthouse.com.

Radiant Heat Saunas

As you know from chapter 6 on Detoxification, sweating is one of the ways in which nature helps us get rid of the toxins that build up in our bodies. The sauna is one way that we can help that natural process along. Well, the last few years have brought High-Tech advances in the world of saunas that make the experience even more pleasurable and effective—and now you can bring these High-Tech saunas into your home. They are called radiant heat saunas.

Radiant heat, also called infrared energy, heats objects directly without having to heat the air in between. It's the kind of heat you get from the sun without its harmful ultraviolet rays.

Traditional saunas use a metal stove, rocks, and a red-hot electric element to heat the air temperature from 180 to 220 degrees Fahrenheit. This superheated air is often uncomfortable. Radiant heat saunas use ceramic heaters that produce air temperatures of 110 to 140 degrees Fahrenheit. However, the radiant heat reaches deeper into the cells of your body while producing two to three times more sweat than other saunas.

Radiant saunas help dilate blood vessels, which improves circulation and strengthens the cardiovascular system. They can also help ease joint pain and stiffness, improve skin tone, and reduce stress and fatigue. And all in the comfort of your own home! These freestanding units come in a variety of sizes, styles, and prices and can be set up indoors or outdoors. Two sources I found were Health Mate saunas from PLH Products, 800-946-6001, and Soft Heat saunas from www.poolproducts.com, 800-983-7665.

Far Infrared Products

Everything on earth absorbs infrared light as heat energy, and it can be captured in many ways to maximize its beneficial qualities. NASA pioneered research into the uses of far infrared technology, which led certain companies into developing products that can have a profound effect on the way people feel. Fibers can be injected with special, light-energized bioceramic powder and can be woven into wraps for different parts of the body. These High-Tech processes provide a safe, natural way of supplying warmth and climate control for our bodies. They also allow the body to perform more effectively in many ways; for instance, infrared light energy breaks large water molecules into smaller ones, releasing trapped toxins in the process. That's why it works well in the sauna. It also warms and expands clogged capillaries, improving circulation. You can find infrared products in heating pads and in wraps for the knees, wrists, and ankles. The wraps radiate far infrared energy through their special ceramic-coated fibers, thereby gently but deeply warming the injury site. You can also get far infrared shower filters, which combine the benefits of water filtration technology with infrared light emissions—useful for preventing mold and soap scum buildup on shower walls.

You can get more information on infrared products by going to www.alternativemedicine.com and reading their article "Warming Up to Far-Infrared." For products, check out a site called www.alkalife.com.

The Far Infrared Hair Dryer

The most popular infrared device in the United States is a hair dryer, marketed under the brand Solride. It prevents hair damage from direct heating—which means fewer split ends and less frizz. It dries hair fibers from the inside out. The infrared heat also penetrates the scalp, increasing blood circulation and helping to remove toxins. The hair dryer has other benefits as well. It is increasingly being used in localized treatments of chronic joint pain and skin conditions (as always, don't use any product until you've spoken to your doctor about it). Some studies have shown that it also helps decrease inflammation and swelling in soft tissue injuries. You can find the Solride at many sites on the Internet, including www.alkalife.com, www.shengoc.kr, and www.selfcare.com.

Cool Stuff for Your Environment

Full-Spectrum Lighting

Dr. John Ott, a world-renowned time-lapse photographer, discovered the benefits of full-spectrum lighting while shooting time-lapse pictures for a movie. According to recent studies, Americans spend nearly 90 percent of their time under artificial light. Full-spectrum lights mimic daylight and cast a true, clear light that soothes tired eyes. Sunlight is composed of many wavelengths of light—some we can see and some we can't. We can see the colors of the rainbow, but we generally can't see ultraviolet or infrared wavelengths. Most regular lightbulbs don't contain all the wavelengths in the visible range. Fluorescent bulbs burn cooler than regular bulbs, but they still do not produce full-spectrum light. A true full-spectrum bulb includes all wavelengths. Full-spectrum lighting provides sharp, consistent visibility and true colors that may lighten your mood, counteract eyestrain and headaches, and encourage a distinct feeling of well-being.

There are hundreds of sources for full-spectrum lights. Two that I recommend are the Cutting Edge catalog (800-497-9516, or www.cutcat.com) and the Tools for Exploration catalog (800-456-9887, or www.toolsforexploration.com).

SAD Lights

According to the National Institute of Mental Health, an estimated thirty-five million Americans suffer from "winter blues," a form of depression that hits during the winter months due to lack of sunlight. Symptoms include lethargy, difficulty concentrating, difficulty waking in the morning, social withdrawal, and irritability. This is known as seasonal affective disorder, commonly called SAD. Natural bright light stimulates the pineal gland, which suppresses the secretion of melatonin, a sleep hormone commonly overproduced by SAD sufferers. It has been estimated that in northern latitudes, this disorder affects up to one in five people.

The standard treatment for SAD is light therapy. That consists of exposure for about thirty minutes a day to full-spectrum lights. There are many light therapy products on the market. One particularly attractive and effective brand is the Happy Lite Light Bath from the Harmony catalog, as well as the Winter Bright Light Box, also available from the Harmony catalog (800-869-3446, or www.gaiam.com) or the True Full-Spectrum SAD-Lite from Tools for Exploration.

HEPA Air Filters

One unfortunate result of technology in today's world is that the air is full of pollutants. It's almost impossible to escape, no matter where you live. Of course, some areas of the country are more polluted than others, but almost everyone is affected—especially children and seniors. In fact, the Department of Consumer Affairs has said that children are more likely to be affected by indoor-air pollution because they breathe faster and inhale more air per unit of body weight than adults. They also warn that the elderly, asthmatics, people with allergies, and people with lung diseases are particularly sensitive to polluted indoor air. High-efficiency particulate arrestance (HEPA) filters can noticeably improve the quality of your indoor air by removing pollen, odors, tobacco smoke, dust, and many other irritants and allergens.

Two sources I recommend are the Healthmate HEPA Air Filter from the Harmony catalog, and the Miracle Air HEPA Air Filtration System from www.pure-natural.com.

Negative Air Ionizers

Negative air ionizers are designed to generate negative ions to re-create the proper atmospheric balance of negative to positive ions. Pollution, synthetic fibers, and electrical devices create positive ions, which then predominate in the air. Negative air ionizers work to rebalance the environment and reduce pollution. The negative ions combine with dust and smoke particles and reverse their polarity so that they drop to the nearest surface. Negative ionizers create a more "normal" environment, almost like being in the fresh air of the country, with a proper balance of negative to positive ions.

Negative ions are attracted to airborne particles, which is how they clean the air—by attracting to particles of dust, pollen, smoke, or dirt and dragging them to the ground. This is something that everyone, especially those who live in cities or more urban areas, should have.

You can find negative air ionizers everywhere, but I recommend the Plasma-Pure from Tools for Exploration, the Elanra Mark II from the Cutting Edge catalog, the Ionix Breeze Quadra Silent Air Purifier from the Sharper Image catalog, or the Surround Air Ionizer from www.surroundair.com. Then there's my personal favorite, the Sani-Mate Ionic Sanilyser, which is specifically designed to control the growth of microscopic bacteria in the bathroom. This one is available from the TechnoScout catalog.

Water Filtration Systems

Water quality is becoming a major problem around the country. You can purchase water analysis kits that can give you information about the various pollutants in your water. That will make it easier for you to find a product that is most appropriate for your needs. There is a wide variety of systems designed to filter water from individual faucets, as well as whole-house systems. There are water ionizers, water distillers, water filters . . . too many to go into. Check out all the catalogs mentioned here to get an idea of what's available.

This is just a sampling of the cool stuff that's out there. The fun part is that technology is advancing so rapidly, in so many directions, there's no telling what will be available tomorrow. I wish the World's Fair would come back to Flushing Meadow; I can't wait to see what visions of the new High-Tech future might contain.

Appendix B:
The Five Pillars Updated

What's new and improved

The world is changing more than any of us could imagine. Humankind, as always, forges ahead through even the worst of times. So, too, does the High-Tech world.

Once again I've chosen to highlight a sampling of some of the new information and products that have come to my attention over the past year within each of the five pillars. They should be added to your arsenal for living your best eighty or ninety years.

Pillar 1: Frontiers

Stem cell therapy continues to evolve. Scientists in Japan have successfully grown the cells of frog eyes and ears, moving closer to the time when we will be able to cultivate organs to replace those that aren't functioning properly. The same doctor who conducted these experiments claims to have grown and successfully transplanted frog kidneys.

In America, Dr. Michael D. West has been conducting experiments in what he calls "human therapeutic cloning." His aim is not to create whole new human beings, but to create parts for existing ones. "I believe we have found the time machine. It is somatic cell nuclear transfer, otherwise known as cloning. . . . We would take a somatic cell from a patient and transfer it into an egg cell whose DNA had been removed. The egg cell would then act as the time machine by taking the patient's cell back to an embryonic state." With this process the embryonic cell would be identical to the patient's own cells, therefore eliminating the risk of rejection.

Although we are still a long way from being able to create spare parts whenever we need them, progress is being made. Dr. West also notes that cloning is "largely trial and error, because we don't know how it works, ultimately. It's magic, it's a black box." In addition, the serious search for an anti-aging pill continues. For many years the most effective way of slowing down aging and increasing life span has been by restricting and reducing calorie consumption. Calorie restriction diets, typically known as CRON (Calorie Restriction Optimum Nutrition), have been practiced on two species of primates in long-term studies. The results concluded that the animals on the CRON diet versus those in the control group survived longer and lived in better health through their later years. One of the measures of this was that they retained more youthful levels of certain hormones, such as the DHEAs that tend to fall with age. The data and research on the CRON diet and its results are extensive. Science is now trying to find a drug or chemical that mimics the effects of the CRON diet on the human body. The best-studied candidate for this kind of agent is called 2DG (2 Deoxy-D-Glucose). This is the future in anti-aging drug development.

Pillar 2: Supernutrition

Every day, the war against obesity continues. Scientists are in hot pursuit of the solution that will help us eat less and burn more fat. Many drug companies are focusing on ways to burn more energy without having to get up off the couch. They're looking at a process called uncoupling. Geoff Watts explains: "the body captures the chemical energy in food by coupling the breakdown of sugar, fat, and protein molecules to the production of ATP, the universal fuel for processes within the cell. ATP then powers the chemical reactions needed to move, think, and do everything else in life. Any leftover ATP is used to produce fat, which is stored within the fat cells throughout the body. Uncoupling allows the body's cells to break down food without creating ATP, effectively flaring off the excess food energy as heat."

There is a family of proteins known as UCPs that are uncoupling proteins. The idea is to design drugs that will persuade the body to make more of these proteins, or to get the ones you already have to work harder. In fact, scientists now believe that natural variations in UCP activity help some people stay thin—no matter what they eat—and others gain weight seemingly just by opening the refrigerator door. Scientists are learning more about how these proteins work and what other processes in the body could be upset by increasing their production or effectiveness. Drugs that work on these proteins would have to be taken for life, and right now we don't know about the long-term effects. So research continues, with a lot of hope and uncertainty.

On the other side of the fence the fast-food industry continues to make a low-fat, healthy way of eating more difficult. More and more nufoods are being introduced every day. The fast-food restaurants around the corner are trying harder to satisfy the country's hunger—or are they, in fact, trying to make us hungrier? There is one ingredient in fast foods that I didn't mention earlier, trans fatty acids. Trans fatty acids are found in hydrogenated oils, the oils to which hydrogen has been added artificially to make them solid and to extend shelf life. The process of hydrogenating fat causes the molecular structure to change into what becomes trans fatty acid. Trans fatty acids are found in many foods, including margarine, some baked goods, and most fast-food products. We've known for many years that trans fatty acid lowers the level of HDL (the good cholesterol) and raises the level of LDL (the bad cholesterol), thus increasing the risks of heart disease. But new studies indicate that the consumption of trans fatty acid on a regular basis alters brain performance where appetite is concerned, actually increasing cravings for sweet and fatty foods. Trans fatty acids also deliver high-density packets of free radicals and increase levels of homocysteine in the body.

The reasons to avoid trans fatty acids just keep growing. It's not always easy to tell when a product contains trans fatty acid, however, or just how much is in the food we eat. So the best defense is simply to lower the overall fat content of your diet—a basic requirement of the Paleotech eating plan.

Nutraceuticals

Before I get into specific new nutraceuticals on the market I want to tell you about a great new company that offers nutraceuticals tailored to your needs. Nutrophy, Inc., a company out of Florida, is creating innovative customized nutritional solutions by incorporating the internet and science technology. Nutrophy, Inc., is a simple yet powerful approach to customizing supplementation in your own home. You begin by filling out an on-line questionnaire at the website (www.nutrophy.com). A computer expert system—Nex, developed in cooperation with some of the top nutritional scientists in the field today—then makes personalized supplement recommendations based on your profile.

Nutrophy has designed a complete array of "no compromise," top-of-the-line supplements using only the best ingredients in the industry. I am very familiar with these, as I was consulted to help create the nutrient combinations and the system itself. It does not end there; once you are a member, the system continues to interact with you via E-mail, delivering personalized content on diet, exercise, and other health-related topics. You can even submit body fluids in the form of saliva and urine for a more accurate and complete profile. The daily supplements are delivered in very cool individualized pouches that fit easily into your lifestyle.

Catch a glimpse of *the future of nutrition* at their website: www.nutrophy.com.

There are some new and highly effective nutraceuticals out on the market. Remember that it is always important to read through the information, find products that apply to your individual needs, and discuss them with your health care provider. Some of the latest developments that are noteworthy include:

Imm-Kine by Allergy Research Group

This is a potent immune system stimulator, which helps maintain healthy cellular growth and inhibits angiogenesis (the growth of blood vessels that are found in cancerous tissue).

VascuStatin by Allergy Research Group

This is also a potent immune system stimulator and angiogenesis inhibitor. Its main ingredient is a leaf extract of bindweed, a plant that has been traditionally used by Native Americans to treat skin ulcers, reducing wound inflammation and swelling.

Oxydrene by Klein-Becker USA

This is a blend of three herbs (*sedum crenulata, hippophae,* and *fructus lychii chinensis*) clinically proven to increase oxygen saturation in blood and tissue. It is designed to maximize your body's ability to build muscle, reduce fat, and increase energy, stamina, and endurance. It can be used by bodybuilders who want to promote muscle growth or by dieters who want to speed up fat loss.

DIM by IAS Limited

DIM is Di-indolylmethane, a phytochemical found in vegetables such as brussels sprouts, broccoli, and cabbage, known to have potent anticancer properties. This product comes in both oral and injectable forms, but right now is available only in Europe and through the internet (see Resource Guide).

Fruits of Life by Garden of Life

This is a 100 percent natural blend of powerful antioxidants, including raspberries, strawberries, raisins, blackberries, and goat's milk in a base of biologically active minerals, enzymes, and probiotics. It's excellent for fighting and neutralizing free radical damage in the body. It comes in powder form; add one teaspoon to one tablespoon to the shakes recommended in chapter 5.

Calcium EAP by Dr. Franz Köhler Chemie, GmbH

This product is currently used in Europe, in both oral and injectable forms, for all diseases that arise from an allergic or autoimmunological process (for example, gastritis, colitis, dermatitis, and eczema). It has also been shown to be effective for certain symptoms of multiple sclerosis.

Infra Therapist by BNH Corporation

This is the latest addition to the category of High-Tech saunas for effective detoxification. It's a truly personal sauna made of fiber-reinforced plastics shaped like an inflated sleeping bag, and it's small enough to be used at home.

MediClear by Thorne Research

This is a rice protein powder with added vitamins, minerals, and nutrients that is an effective addition to your detoxification routine. It is useful in treating poor digestion, allergies, inflammation, blood sugar abnormalities, and certain hormone imbalances.

Oz Garcia's Longevity Pack and System, by Oz Garcia

Up to this point, I've had no financial stake in any of the products I've recommended. In the interest of full disclosure, however (and as you can probably guess by the name), I will say that this is a new product line I have developed to make it easier for you to get the nutrients you need for each pillar—in one convenient packet. This anti-aging, life-extension longevity pack contains five pills to be taken on a daily basis. Each pill contains its own individual set of nutrients:

1. A perfect combination of essential fatty acids, including DHA and omega-3 fatty acids

2. A blend of antioxidants to reduce the effects of premature aging

3. A brain-power formula designed to produce amplification of mental capacities

4. A blend of MSM, silica, and hyaluronic acid for healthier, younger-looking skin and hair

5. A hormone regulator for both men and women

Cosmeceuticals

On the cosmeceutical front there are new and innovative products that improve quality of skin by improving collagen synthesis in an extraordinary and unique manner. These human-placenta-based products also make hair grow. I discovered them while traveling through Russia. They are from a patented and highly studied extract of human placenta called Plazan. Based on my research, I feel that this product is at the beginning of the next generation of cosmeceuticals. It comes in a variety of forms such as facial masks, face and body creams, shampoos, and balms. These products place the placenta stem cell right where it is needed—on the surface of your skin and at the aging hair follicle site. They are currently available on our website, www.ozgarcia.com, and through my office.

Pillar 3: Life Extension, Life Enhancement

The future of individualized medicine—the ability to diagnose and treat disease on a case-by-case basis—has gone a step further. The Great Smokies Diagnostic Laboratory developed Genovations™, a system of testing an individual patient's unique genetic predisposition. By testing either blood or saliva samples, Genovations can identify gene defects that contribute to chronic diseases such as asthma, autoimmune disorders, certain cancers, allergies, infectious diseases, arthritis, heart disease, and stroke. Physicians armed with such early warning signs can use more precise and more customized interventions—earlier—while helping patients modify diet and exercise and prescribing the most helpful drugs and/or nutraceuticals. While this is a tremendous breakthrough in the prevention and treatment of many diseases, it is important to remember that these tests can indicate only risk, not certainty. Testing positive for a gene defect doesn't mean that you are sure to develop a health problem. And if you don't have a particular gene defect, it doesn't mean that you are guaranteed protection from getting that disease. However, knowing your own personal susceptibilities can be of great benefit in developing a lifestyle for a long and healthy life.

Research continues in all areas of life extension and enhancement. For instance, telemedicine (see chapter 1) is becoming more and more of a reality. A new NASA-sponsored system recently helped a team of surgeons in Japan remove a fibroid tumor from a woman without removing her uterus. The Japanese surgeons were helped by a team of doctors in America using an instant MRI—powerful computerized imaging from inside the body seen simultaneously by both the American and the Japanese doctors.

European cell treatments continue to be ahead of the curve, as they are beginning to use undifferentiated human stem cells in place of the animal products previously used. In Eastern Europe and in India clinics are beginning to offer treatments using both umbilical stem cells and adult marrow stem cells. Laws will likely prevent these treatments from being available in the Western world for a long time to come, but the technology that makes them possible continues to advance rapidly in other parts of the world.

Also from Eastern Europe comes another breakthrough discovery: the use of NAC (n-acetylcarnosine) eyedrops to cure—and prevent—cataracts. This treatment has been used successfully in Russia and China, but is not common in America. In a clinical trial in Russia, these eyedrops were used to treat ninety-six cataract patients, age sixty and above. Each patient was treated with one to two drops into each eye three times a day for up to six months. All of the patients showed marked improvement with no side effects. It is also believed that use of this product can prevent the first occurrence of cataracts.

Pillar 4: The Body Beautiful

There's a new name in town when it comes to the Body Beautiful: Mésothérapie, a medical specialty that was developed in France by Dr. Michel Pistor in the early fifties. Mésothérapie stimulates the mesoderm (the middle layer of the skin) and is used to eliminate cellulite and wrinkles, to tone the skin, and to treat hair loss, pain, psoriasis, migraines, and allergies.

The process involves injecting compounds made of various pharmacological agents, plant extracts, vitamins, and minerals into the skin at the place of treatment. The ingredients vary according to the problem being treated, but generally fall into categories like anti-inflammatories, muscle relaxants, anti-infectants, hormones, hormone blockers, and anesthetics. The injections are made with tiny needles that don't penetrate the skin very deeply.

Right now there are more than 15,000 practitioners of Mésothérapie in France alone, and many others around the world. However, there are currently only about fifteen specialists in the United States, though that number is growing quickly. One of the foremost practitioners here is Dr. Lionel Bissoon, the American consultant for the International Course on Mésothérapie.

"Although Mésothérapie can be used medicinally for such ailments as rheumatoid arthritis and migraines," says Dr. Bissoon, "most of my practice involves retarding the aging process. For instance, Mésothérapie can be used to stimulate hair growth in men and women. It is also very effective in reducing cellulite and eliminating lines around the eyes and the mouth. Its most dramatic results are for tightening loose skin around the neck and for rejuvenating hands that are beginning to show signs of aging. Nothing can stop the aging process, but Mésothérapie can certainly slow it down and help the skin continue to look youthful and resilient."

Pillar 5: Sexuality

The debate over hormone replacement treatments continues. For the past several decades, the medical community has made many assumptions about HRT that are proving to be false. While HRT's drawbacks were well known (including increased risks of blood clots and breast cancer), claims have been made that in addition to relieving symptoms such as hot flashes and night sweats, HRT could also prevent or treat a variety of ailments in postmenopausal women, including heart disease, osteoporosis, depression, urinary incontinence, and Alzheimer's disease.

But a new study in the *Internal Position Paper on Women's Health and Menopause* proves that the medical community has been wrong. The paper shows that instead of protecting women from heart attacks and stroke, HRT has increased their risk. In fact, there was a 50 percent increase in the risk of heart attacks in the first year of HRT treatment in women who already had heart disease. Another study showed a significant increase in the risk of stroke for women taking HRT. Clinical trials have shown no benefit as far as Alzheimer's disease is concerned, and while HRT can prevent bone loss from osteoporosis, the bone loss resumes as soon as the medication is stopped.

Dr. Erika Schwartz, author of *The Hormone Solution*, is squarely on the side of natural hormone treatments. For women who complain of lack of libido or sexual discomfort, she recommends specially formulated micronized testosterone creams applied to the clitoris and inner labia before sex. The results are remarkable, and according to Dr. Schwartz, "no one complains of growing whiskers or developing baritone voices." In addition, Dr. Schwartz says that it's important to rebalance hormones that are causing these symptoms, "Natural progesterone and estradiol combined will bring back your flagging sex drive."

Getting these hormones involves a visit to a knowledgeable, interested doctor who is willing and able to write a prescription for you and knows where to get the best-quality natural hormones. Keep in mind that these creams are individually mixed, so the quality of the product depends on the experience of the pharmacy you're getting it from.

One place I recommend is the Natural Hormone Pharmacy, a New York State–based specialty compounding pharmacy (see Resource Guide) that has developed an over-the-counter cream made from the amino acid L-arginine, which, when applied right before sex, produces increased blood flow to the clitoris.

As far as other symptoms of menopause, Dr. Schwartz says: "Once you connect the symptom—hot flashes, insomnia, night sweats, depression, bloating, weight gain, migraines, etc., to hormone imbalance, you can approach the situation correctly. Your hormones need to be replenished. This doesn't mean you need synthetic hormone replacement. You just need to supplement hormones you're missing, and you can do that with natural hormones.

"Natural hormones are read by the human body as part of its own. Administered in a medically supervised manner, natural hormones can safely treat the root cause of hormonal imbalances and deficiencies, and their attendant symptoms. The result? A younger, healthier you."

I could go on and on—if I only had the time and space in this book—but this is health we are talking about. More specifically, the high-tech future of health, so it is by definition an ongoing topic. It's now up to you to stay curious and keep an open mind for a long, long, healthy life.

Resource Guide

The following companies make high-quality products that I often use in my practice:

BNH Corporation
7171 Orangethorpe Avenue
Buena Park, CA 90621
Phone: 800-969-9336
www.saunaplus.com

Cytodyne Technologies Inc.
P.O. Box 1421
Lakewood, NJ 08701
Phone: 888-CYTODYN
www.cytodyne.com

Ecological Formulas
1061-B Shary Circle
Concord, CA 94518
Phone: 800-351-9429
Fax: 925-676-9231

Enada Corp.
Menuco Corp.
Phone: 212-736-1039
www.enada.com
www.menuco.com

Garden of Life
1449 Jupiter Park Drive, Suite 16
Jupiter, FL 33458

Phone: 800-688-8986
www.gardenoflifeusa.com

Great Smokies Diagnostic Laboratory
63 Zillicoa Street
Asheville, NC 28801
Phone: 800-522-4762
www.gsdl.com

Healthmate Saunas
16000 Phoenix Drive
City of Industry, CA 91745-1623
Phone: 800-946-6001
Fax: 626-968-0444
www.saunaplus.com

IAS Limited
c/o Les Autelets, Suite I
Sark GY9 OSF
Great Britain
Phone: +44 870 151 4144
Fax: +44 709 211 5519 or
+44 870 151 4145
www.antiaging-systems.com

Klein-Becker USA
402 West 5050 North
Provo, UT 84604
Phone: 888-340-1628

Life Enhancement
P.O. Box 751390
Petaluma, CA 94975-1390
Phone: 800-LIFE-873
www.life-enhancement.com

Life Extension Foundation
1100 West Commercial Boulevard
Fort Lauderdale, FL 33309
Phone: 800-544-4440
www.oz.lef.org

Metagenics
166 Fernwood Avenue
Edison, NJ 08837
Phone: 800-638-2848
Fax: 732-417-1222
www.metagenics.com

Natren Inc.
3105 Willow Lane
Westlake Village, CA 91361
Phone: 800-992-3323
Fax: 805-371-4742
www.natren.com

Natural Hormone Pharmacy
200 Saw Mill River Road
Hawthorne, NY 10532
www.naturalhormonepharmacy.com
Phone: 914-747-1805

Nutraceutics/Pharmalogic
3317 NW 10th Terrace, Suite 404
Fort Lauderdale, FL 33309
Phone: 800-391-0114
Fax: 954-725-3904
www.nutraceutics.com
www.pharmalogic.net
E-mail: ralvarez@pharmalogic.net

Nutricology
(also called Allergy Research)
Allergy Research
30806 Santana Street
Hayward, CA 94544
Phone: 510-487-8526
Toll-free Phone: 800-545-9960
www.allergyresearchgroup.com

Nutrophy, Inc.
7003 N. Waterway Drive
Suite 222
Miami, FL 3 3155
Phone: 305-260-0883
Fax: 305-260-9395
www.nutrophy.com

Skin Biology
12833 SE 40th Place
Bellevue, WA 98006
Phone: 800-405-1912
www.skinbio.com

Thorne Research
25820 Highway 2 West
P.O. Box 25
Dover, ID 83825
Phone: 800-228-1966
Fax: 800-747-1950
www.thorne.com

Twinlabs
150 Motor Parkway, Suite 210
Hauppauge, NY 11788
Phone: 800-645-5626
Fax: 631-630-3488
www.twinlab.com

Uni Key Health Systems Inc.
Uni Key
P.O. Box 7168
Bozeman, MT 59771
Phone: 800-888-4353
Fax: 406-585-9892
www.unikeyhealth.com

**The following publications are excellent
resources for information on nutrition
and supplements:**

Alternative Medicine
1650 Tiburon Boulevard
Tiburon, CA 94920
Phone: 800-546-6707 (subscriptions)
Phone: 800-515-4325
www.alternativemedicine.com

Life Extension
Life Extension Foundation
P.O. Box 229120
Hollywood, FL 33022
Phone: 800-544-4440
www.lef.org

Men's Health
www.menshealth.com
Phone: 800-666-2303

Muscle & Fitness
Muscle & Fitness letters
21100 Erwin Street
Woodland Hills, CA 91367
Phone: 800-340-8954 (subscriptions)
Fax: 818-595-0463
www.muscle-fitness.com

Muscle Media
555 Corporate Circle
Golden, CO 80401
Phone: 800-615-8500

Muscular Development
P.O. Box 765
Medford, NY 11763-9862
Phone: 888-841-8007
www.musculardevelopment.com

*The Townsend Letter for Doctors
and Patients*
911 Tyler Street
Port Townsend, WA 98368-6541

The following are individuals, clinics, societies, and organizations that are excellent sources of information and/or treatment:

Dr. Lionel Bissoon
10 West 74th Street
New York, NY 10023
Phone: 212-579-9136
Anushka Spa
Palm Beach Gardens, FL
Phone: 561-630-5555
www.meso.com

Dr. Stephen Bosniak
122 East 64 Street
New York, NY 10021
Phone: 212-769-0740
www.eye-lift.com

Cenegenics Medical Institute
851 Rampart Boulevard
Las Vegas, NV 89145
Phone: 888-YOUNGER
www.888younger.com

Clinique La Prairie
CH-1815 Clarens
Montreux, Switzerland
Phone: 41(21) 989 33 11
www.laprairie.ch

Dr. Allan Dunn
North Miami Beach Florida
Phone: 888-848-6534

Dr. Richard Firshein
The Firshein Center for
Comprehensive Medicine
1226 Park Avenue
New York, NY 10128
Phone: 212-860-0282
www.DrCity.com
DrFirshein@drcity.com

Ann Louise Gittleman, N.D, M.S., C.N.S.
ALG Inc.
P.O. Box 882
Bozeman, MT 59771
Phone: 704-895-9104
Fax: 704-895-7916
www.annlouise.com
www.flatflush.com
www.ivillage.com/diet/boards

Immune Institute
Dr. Daryl See
18800 Delaware Street, Suite 900
Huntington Beach, CA 92648
Phone: 714-596-8822

International Clinic of
Biological Regeneration
North American Office
P.O. Box 509
Florissant, MO 63032
Phone: 800-826-5366; 314-921-3997

International Society for the Application
of Organ Filtrates, Cellular Therapy,
and Oncobiotherapy
Robert Bosch Strasse, 56a D-6909
Walldorf, Germany
Phone: 0620276-3268
Fax: 062227-6330

Pamela M. Peeke, M.D., M.P.H.
5413 West Cedar Lane
Suite 206C
Bethesda, MD 20814
Phone: 301-897-3333
Fax: 301-414-0300
www.drpeeke.com
www.fightfatafter40.com
The Peeke Newsletter on-line weekly

Dr. Nicholas Perricone
Clinical Creations
35 Pleasant Street, Suite 1C
Meriden, CT 06450
Phone: 888-823-7837
www.clinicalcreations.com
www.nvperriconemd.com

Dr. Peter Proctor
4126 SW Freeway
Suite 1616
Houston, TX 77017
Phone: 713-960-1616
www.drproctor.com

Dr. Ron Ruden
Ruden and Jaffe Associates
201 East 65 Street
New York, NY 10021
Phone: 212-879-4700

Dr. Erika Schwartz
10 West 74th Street
New York, NY 10023
Phone: 212-579-9136

The Stephan Clinic
27 Harley Place, Harley Street
London, England W1N 1HB
Phone: 071-636-6196
Fax: 071-255-1626

University HeartScan
307 East 63 Street
New York, NY 10021
Phone: 212-546-9292

Bibliography

Ainsworth, Claire. "How to Burn Off Blubber Without Moving a Muscle." *New Scientist*. December 2, 2000. www.newscientist.com.

Allport, Susan. *The Primal Feast: Food, Sex, Foraging, and Love*. New York: Harmony Books, 2000.

Arnot, Robert. *Dr. Bob's Revolutionary Weight Control Program*. New York: Little, Brown, 1997.

Associated Press. "Study Focuses on Appetite Signals." *New York Times*. April 11, 2001. www.nytimes.com.

Balch, James F., and Phyllis A. Balch. *Prescription for Nutritional Healing A-to-Z Guide to Supplements*. Garden City Park, NY: Avery Publishing Group, Inc., 1998.

Ball, Eddy, Patrick Runkel, and Scott Homes (editors). *Functional Assessment Resource Manual*. Asheville, SC: Great Smokies Diagnostic Laboratory, 1999.

Berkson, Lindsey D. *Hormone Deception: How Everyday Foods and Products Are Disrupting Your Hormones—and How to Protect Yourself and Your Family*. Chicago: Contemporary Books, 2000.

Brodish, Paul. "The Irreversible Effects of Cigarette Smoking." American Council on Science and Health. www.acsc.org.

Brody, Jane E. "One-Two Punch for Losing Pounds: Exercise and Careful Diet." *New York Times*. October 17, 2000. www.nytimes.com.

Brown, Kathryn. "The Human Genome Business Today." *Scientific American*. July 2000; 50–55.

Chud, Deborah Friedson. *The Gourmet Prescription: High Flavor Recipes for Lower Carbohydrate Diets*. San Francisco: Bay Books, 1999.

Ciarallo, Lydia, M.D., David Brousseau, M.D., and Steven Reinert M.S. "Higher-dose intravenous magnesium therapy for children with moderate to severe acute asthma." *Archives of Pediatrics and Adolescent Medicine*. October 25, 2000; 154:979–983.

Davis, Robert. "The Inside Story: Reporter takes uncertain plunge into his own body." *USA Today.* August 25, 2000. www.usatoday.com.

Dement, William, M.D. *The Promise of Sleep.* New York: Dell Publishing, 1999.

Devanand, D. P., et al. "Olfactory deficits in patients with mild cognitive impairment predict Alzheimer's follow-up." *American Journal of Psychiatry.* September 2000:1399–1405.

Eades, Michael R., and Mary Dan Eades. *Protein Power.* New York: Bantam Books, 1996.

Ellis, F. R., and S. Nasser. "A pilot study of vitamin B_{12} in the treatment of tiredness." *British Journal of Nutrition.* 1973; 30:277–283.

Friedland, Robert P., Thomas Fritsch, Kathleen A. Smyth, et al. "Patients with Alzheimer's disease have reduced activities in midlife compared with healthy control-group members." *Proceedings of the National Academy of Sciences.* March 13, 2001; 98(6):3440–3445.

Fritsch, Jane. "95% Regain Lost Weight. Or Do They?" *New York Times.* May 25, 1999. www.nytimes.com.

Garcia, Oz. *The Balance.* New York: HarperCollins, 1998.

Gard, Zane R., M.D., et al. "Toxic Bio-Accumulation and Effective Detoxification." Human Environmental Medicine, Inc., 1987.

Gardner, Gary, and Brian Halweil. "Chronic Hunger and Obesity Epidemic Eroding Global Progress." Worldwatch Institute. March 4, 2000. www.worldwatch.org.

Gaynor, Mitchell L., M.D., and Jerry Hickey, R.Ph. *Dr. Gaynor's Cancer Prevention Program.* New York: Kensington Books, 1999.

Gittleman, Ann Louise. *Before the Change: Taking Charge of Your Perimenopause.* New York: HarperCollins, 1998.

Gittleman, Ann Louise. *Super Nutrition for Men.* New York: M. Evans and Company, Inc., 1996.

Goggin and Stelmach. *Aging and Cognition: Mental Processes, Self Awareness and Interventions.* Amsterdam: North Holland Press, 1990.

Grady, Denise. "Scientists Question Hormone Therapies for Menopause

Ills." *New York Times.* April 18,2002. www.nytimes.com.

Hegarty, Verona M., Helen M. May, and Kay-Tee Khaw. "Tea drinking and bone mineral density in older women." *American Journal of Clinical Nutrition.* 2000; 71:1003–1007.

Heinonen, O. P., D. Albanes, J. Virtano, P. R. Taylor, J. K. Huttenen, et al. "Prostate cancer and supplementation with alpha-tocopherol and beta-carotene: incidence and mortality in a controlled trial." *Journal of the National Cancer Institute.* March 18, 1998; 90:440–446.

Iso, H., K. M. Rexrode, M. J. Stampfer, J. E. Manson, G. A. Colditz, F. E. Speizer, C. H. Hennekens, and W. C. Willet. "Intake of Fish and Omega-3 Fatty Acids and Risk of Stroke in Women." *Journal of the American Medical Association.* January 17, 2001; 285(3):304–312.

Jamieson, James, Dr. L. E. Dorman, with Valerie Marriott. *Growth Hormone: The Methuselah Factor.* East Canaan, CT: Safe Goods, 1997.

Kaku, Michio. *Visions: How Science Will Revolutionize the 21st Century.* New York: Bantam Books, 1998.

Kant, Ashima K. "Consumption of energy-dense, nutrient-poor foods by adult Americans: nutritional and health implications." *American Journal of Clinical Nutrition.* October 2000; 72(4):929–936.

Kent, Saul. "Therapeutic Cloning Under Fire: An Interview with Michael D. West, Ph.D." *Life Extension.* March 2002; 38–46.

Kirschmann, Gayla J., and John D. Kirschmann. *Nutrition Almanac.* New York: McGraw-Hill, 1996.

Kolata, Gina. "How the Body Knows When to Gain or Lose." *New York Times.* October 17, 2000. www.nytimes.com.

Laino, Charlene. "First gene-modified monkey is born." January 11, 2001. www.msnbc.com.

Lane, Mark A., Donald K. Ingram, and George S. Roth. "The Serious Search for an Anti-Aging Pill." *Scientific American.* August 2002. www.sciam.com.

Leithauser, Brad. "Feeling Better." *Men's Journal.* October 2000; 72–78.

Life Extension Foundation. *The Physician's Guide to Life Extension Drugs.* Fort Lauderdale, FL, 2000.

Lim, Dr. Joyce. "Carbon Dioxide Laser Resurfacing." *NSC Bulletin*. Volume 8, no. 1, 1997. www.nsc.gov.

Linder, Lawrence. "Stone Age Soup." *Washington Post*. February 13, 2001: HE09.

Linos, Athena, Virginia G. Kaklamani, Evangelina Kaklamani, Yvonni Koutmantiaki, Ernestini Giziaki, Sotiris Papzoglou, and Christos S. Mantzoros. "Dietary factors in relation to rheumatoid arthritis: a role for olive oil and cooked vegetables?" *American Journal of Clinical Nutrition*. 1999; 70:1077–1082.

Ludwig, David S., Karen E. Peterson, and Steven L. Gortmaker. "Relation between consumption of sugar-sweetened drinks and childhood obesity: a prospective, observational analysis." *The Lancet*. February 17, 2001; 357:505.

Mallek, Henry, Ph.D. *The New Longevity Diet: How to Stay Young, Stay Healthy, Stay Slim by Eating the Foods You Love*. New York: Putnam Publishing Group, 2000.

Mitchell, Terri. "Reinventing the Brain." *Life Extension*. August 2000. www.oz.lef.org/magazine.

Mooney, David J., and Antonios G. Mikos. "Growing New Organs." *Scientific American Presents*. November 1999; 10–15.

MSNBC. "Nano-technology makes giant strides." May 18, 2000. www.msnbc.com.

National Institutes of Health. "Stem Cells: A Primer." May 2000. www.nih.gov.

Paw, M. J., N. de Jong, E. G. Pallast, G. C. Kloek, E. G. Schouten, and F. J. Kok. "Immunity in frail elderly: a randomized controlled trial of exercise and enriched foods." *Medicine and Science in Sports and Exercise*. December 2000; 32(12):2005–2011.

Peeke, Pamela M. *Fight Fat After Forty*. New York: Viking Press, 2000.

Perlmutter, Dr. David. *Brainrecovery.com*. Naples, FL: David Perlmutter, 2000.

Perricone, Nicholas. *The Wrinkle Cure: Unlock the Power of Cosmeceuticals for Supple, Youthful Skin*. Emmaus, PA: Rodale Books, 2000.

Pescovitz, David. "Spare parts for vital organs." *Scientific American Presents*. September 2000; 62–67.

Regaldo, Antonio. "Alzheimer's Vaccine Shows Promise in Test." *Wall Street Journal.* December 21, 2000; 35.

Renehan, Edward. *Scientific American Guide to Science on the Internet.* New York: Simon & Schuster, 2000.

Ridker, Paul M., M.D., Julie E. Buring, Sc.D., et al. "Prospective study of C-Reactive Protein and the risk of future cardiovascular events among apparently healthy women." *Circulation.* 1998; 98: 731–733.

Rouhianen, P., H. Rouhiainen, and J. T. Salonen. "Association between low plasma vitamin E concentration and progression of early cortical lens opacities." *American Journal of Epidemiology.* 1996; 144(5): 496–500.

Schwartz, Erika, M.D. *The Hormone Solution: Naturally Alleviate Symptoms of Hormone Imbalance from Adolescence Through Menopause.* New York: Warner Books, Inc., 2002.

Segala, Melanie (editor). *Disease Prevention and Treatment.* Fort Lauderdale, FL: Life Extension Foundation, 2000.

Sheats, Cliff. *Lean Bodies.* New York: Warner Books, 1995.

Shnare, Denk, Shields, and Brunton. "Evaluation of a detoxification regimen for fat stored Zenobiotics." *Medical Hypotheses.* 1982; 9.

Simontacchi, Carol. *The Crazy Makers: How the Food Industry Is Destroying Our Brains and Harming Our Children.* New York: Penguin Putnam Inc., 2000.

Sinatra, Dr. Stephen. *Heart Sense for Women.* Washington, DC: Lifeline Press, 2000.

Sinha, Gunjan. "The Doctor Is in the House." *Popular Science.* July 2000; 50–54.

Smith, Carol. "Genome Q&A." *Seattle Post-Intelligencer.* June 27, 2000. http://seattlep-i.nwsource.com.

Smith, Wayne, Paul Mitchell, and Stephen R. Leeder. "Dietary Fat and Fish Intake and Age-Related Maculopathy." *Archives of Ophthalmology.* 2000; 188:401–404.

Stolz, Craig. "Health Talk: Healthy Aging." *Washington Post.* April 18, 2000. www.washingtonpost.com.

Time Inc Health. *The Healing Power of SuperFoods.* San Francisco: Time Health Media, Inc., 1999.

Van Cauter, Eve, Ph.D., Rachel Leproult, M.S., and Laurence Plat, M.D. "Age-Related Changes in Slow Wave Sleep and REM Sleep and Relationship with Growth Hormone and Cortisol Levels in Healthy Men." *Journal of the American Medical Association.* August 16, 2000; 284:861.

Verhoef, P., et al. "Plasma total homocysteine, B vitamins, and risk of coronary atherosclerosis." *Arteriosclerosis, Thrombosis, and Vascular Biology.* 1997; 17: 989–995.

Wade, Nicholas. "Teaching the Body to Heal Itself." *New York Times.* November 7, 2000. www.nytimes.com.

Wang, Gene-Jack, Nora D. Volkow, Jean Logan, Noami R. Pappas, Christopher T. Wong, Wei Zhu, Noelwah Netusil, and Joanna S. Fowlder. "Brain dopamine and obesity." *The Lancet.* February 2001; 357: 354–357.

Watts, George. "Dig In, Dine On, Pig Out." *New Scientist.* March 2002; 29–32.

Weinblatt, Dr. Michael E. *The Arthritis Action Program: An Integrated Plan of Traditional and Complementary Therapies.* New York: Simon & Schuster, 2000.

Wetzel, Miriam S., Ph.D., David M. Eisenberg, M.D., and Ted J. Kaptchuck, O.M.D. "Courses involving complementary and alternative medicine at US medical schools." *Journal of the American Medical Association.* September 2, 1998; 280(9): 784–787.

Williamson, David. "New research finds link between gum disease, acute heart attacks." November 12, 2000. www.eurekalert.org

Zheng, W., T. J. Doyle, L. H. Kushi, T. A. Sellers, C. P. Hong, and A. R. Folsom. "Tea consumption and cancer incidence in a prospective cohort study of postmenopausal women." *American Journal of Epidemiology.* 1996; 144:175–182.

Zorpette, Glenn. "Muscular Again." *Scientific American Presents Your Bionic Future.* November 22, 1999; 27–31.

Index

acetylcholine, 137, 138, 139, 200–201, 202

acetylcholinesterase (AchE), 200–201

acetyl-L-carnitine (ALC), 138, 141, 142, 196

adenosine di-phosphate (ADP), 288

adenosine tri-phosphate (ATP), 138, 146, 199, 288

adenovirus-36, 109–10

adrenal glands, 43, 119, 151

adult stem cells, 27–28

Advanced Glycatian End Products (AGEs), 55, 130, 186, 189

alcohol, 7, 34, 133, 161

Allport, Susan, 164

Aloe Seltzer C, 154–55

alpha-carotene, 46

alpha-hydroxy acids (AHA), 266, 267–68

alpha lipoic acid (ALA), 263, 265, 266

Alpha MSH (PT-141), 307

Alprostadil, 307

Alzheimer's disease, 6, 46, 48–49, 57, 137, 139, 151, 156, 178, 187, 189, 190, 200–204, 214, 251–52

aminexil, 281–82

amino acids, 42, 57–58, 132, 138, 145–46, 155, 198–99, 283, 289

see also specific amino acids

Amino Acids Analysis, 242–43

anchovies, green bean–tomato salad with tuna, olives and, 80–81

androderm, 304

andropause, 11, 224, 300, 302–5

Angier, Natalie, 312

antibiotics, 54, 55, 133, 238

antibodies, 25, 203, 217

antidepressants, 132, 157

antigens, 25, 217

antioxidants, 6, 40, 45, 47, 53, 54, 192, 262, 264

detoxification and, 165, 166, 175

nutraceuticals as, 131, 133, 135, 139

anxiety, 4, 48, 57, 137, 140, 155

ApoEe-4 gene, 202, 203

Appage, Thierry Pache, 315

apple(s), 47

creamed trout toasts with, 70

apricot(s), 162

cream, mixed berry bowl with, 67

Apomorphine (Uprima), 307–8

arachidonic acid, 189, 266

arterial system, 10, 49, 58, 130, 234, 249

arthritis, 11, 50, 131, 157, 238, 294–97

see also osteoarthritis

asparagus:

garlic, shrimp marinara with, 87

roasted garlic, 88

asthma, 208, 209, 214

avocado-ginger sauce, crab bundles with, 81–82

bacopa monniera extract, 140

Bailey, Covert, 116

balsamic:

grilled lamb chops, 84

vinaigrette, basic, 65

barley:

chicken, and mushroom soup, hearty, 76–77

-oatmeal cakes, 72–73

Barr, Ronald, 114

bean(s), 69

black, huevos rancheros with, 68–69

in buffalo chili, 100–101

green, –tomato salad with tuna, anchovies, and olives, 80–81

chicken, and barley soup, hearty,
78–79
portobello, "pizzas," 76
mustard dressing, grainy, cold chicken and cauliflower salad with, 82–83
Myers cocktail, 208–12
Myoplex, 121, 135

NAC eyedrops, 340
NADH (reduced B-nicotinamide adenine dinucleotide), 121, 139
nail care, 272–73
nanotechnology, 2, 20–21
NatCell, 219
National Institute on Aging (NIA), 8, 190
Natren intestinal bacteria, 134
negative air ionizers, 328–29
nerve growth factor (NGF), 200, 202–3
nettles, 305
neurotoxins, *see* excitotoxins
neurotransmitters, 137, 138, 139, 170, 181–82, 186,
195–96, 198
niacin (vitamin B$_3$), 171–72, 239
Niehans, Paul, 215, 217, 218
Nielsen, Jerri, 16, 17
90-Day Healthy High-Tech Body Program,
317–21
nitric oxide, 198
Nizoral, 281, 282
nonsteroidal anti-inflammatory drugs (NSAIDs),
190–91, 202, 295, 296
nootropics (smart drugs), 178, 185, 192, 196–201,
211–12
noradrenaline, 57
Northrup, Christiane, 312, 314
nuclear factor kappa B (NFkB), 260–61, 263
nucleotides, 53
nufood, 37–38, 112
Nurses Health Study, 46, 314
nutraceuticals, 6, 35–36, 126–59, 335–38
for brain, 136–41
fitness and, 287–88
injectable, 207–14

sexuality and, 304–5
for skin and hair, 263–64
weight control and, 112, 120–23, 126
Nutraceutics, 149–50, 154–55
Nutricology, 124, 130, 133–36, 138, 199
nuts, facts about, 48

oatmeal-barley cakes, 72–73
OKG, 146, 289
olive oil, 48, 49, 51, 238, 295–96
olives, green bean–tomato salad with tuna,
anchovies, and, 80–81
omega-3 fatty acids, 40, 45, 47–50, 60, 166, 262,
265
DHA, 48–49, 136
onion(s):
and leek "pizzas," breakfast, 73
Vidalia, pork tenderloin smothered with
grapes and, 89–90
organs, cloning of, 4, 14
organ transplants, 23–26
osteoarthritis, 157, 158, 265, 294, 296–97
osteoporosis, 130, 236, 244, 245, 248
Ott, John, 327

Paleotech Diet, 4–5, 35, 37–58, 189, 262
enhancers for, 53–55
hormones and, 41–45, 49
principles of, 39–41, 45, 111
Paleotech Gourmet, 5, 35, 59–103
pancreas, 51, 57
pap smear, 234
parathyroid blocking compounds, 283
Parkinson's disease, 57, 139, 168, 178, 187, 213
Pearson, Dirk, 199
Peeke, Pamela, xiii, 312, 315
Pelton, Ross, 197
pepper, frittata with garlic chives, 71
peppers, roasted, broccoli rabe with tomatoes and,
86
perifollicular fibrosis, 281–82
perimenopause, 150, 310, 311, 312
periodontal disease, 10, 240

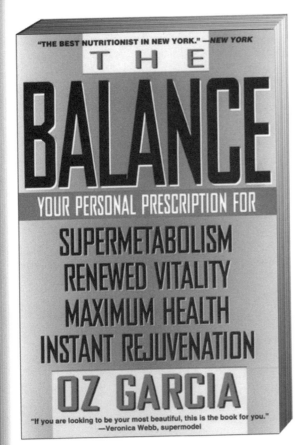
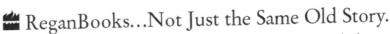

Longevity: your solution to successful aging

Introducing a complete nutraceutical package
for all your anti-aging needs

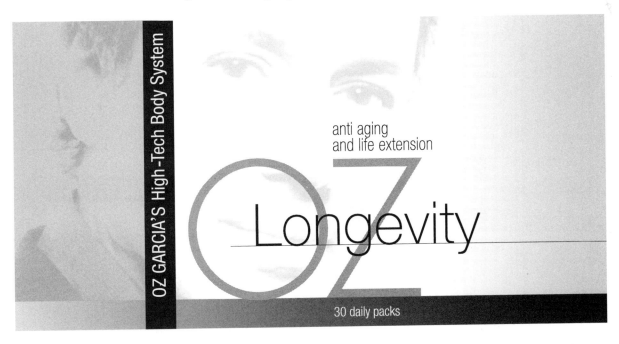

anti aging
and life extension

OZ GARCIA'S High-Tech Body System

OZ Longevity

30 daily packs

An antidote to premature aging, this powerful and innovative supplement pack, taken once a day, returns your health to maximum efficiency.

Follow the guidelines of *Look and Feel Fabulous Forever* and add Longevity to your routine to:

- Control wrinkling and erase the signs of external aging
- Undo the damages of free radicals, glycation, and inflammation
- Experience hormonal revitalization
- Noticeably improve your moods and dramatically increase energy
- Build new and healthy brain performance
- Build a strong immunological defense against degenerative illness

Based on over three years of intensive research and development, Longevity is innovative, scientifically sound, and medically endorsed by top doctors and researchers.

Call Longevity now to order your thirty-day supply

To order, call 866-252-5980 ext. 2990 or online at www.ozgarcia.com

Not sponsored or endorsed by HarperCollins Publishers

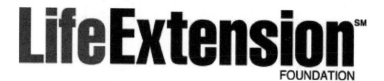
LifeExtension^{SM}
FOUNDATION

Knowledge Base CD-ROM

A compilation of research, treatments, and indispensable information is contained on this FREE CD-ROM (a $24.95 retail value).

❏ An interactive version of Life Extension's 945-page reference volume, *Disease Prevention and Treatment,* which provides information on 118 diseases and health conditions. These innovative medical therapies are used to treat degenerative diseases of aging, including heart disease, cancer, stroke, Alzheimer's disease, and more.

❏ An archive of articles from the last year of *Life Extension* magazine. We have included articles such as "Antioxidant Power," "How CoQ10 Protects Your Cardiovascular System," "How Men Can Safely Use Testosterone to Restore Libido," and "Enhancing Cognitive Function."

❏ Healthy and delicious **RECIPES** from Oz Garcia—exclusively on the CD-ROM. Convenient one-page format allows you to print a recipe and take it with you while food shopping or E-mail it to friends. Eat well!

❏ Useful links to **OzGarcia.com,** the website of a world authority on nutrition and wellness and the author of *Look and Feel Fabulous Forever,* LifeExtension.com, and HarperCollins.com.

Use the postcard in this copy of *Look and Feel Fabulous Forever* to obtain your Life Extension Knowledge Base CD-ROM today!